massage
mind and body

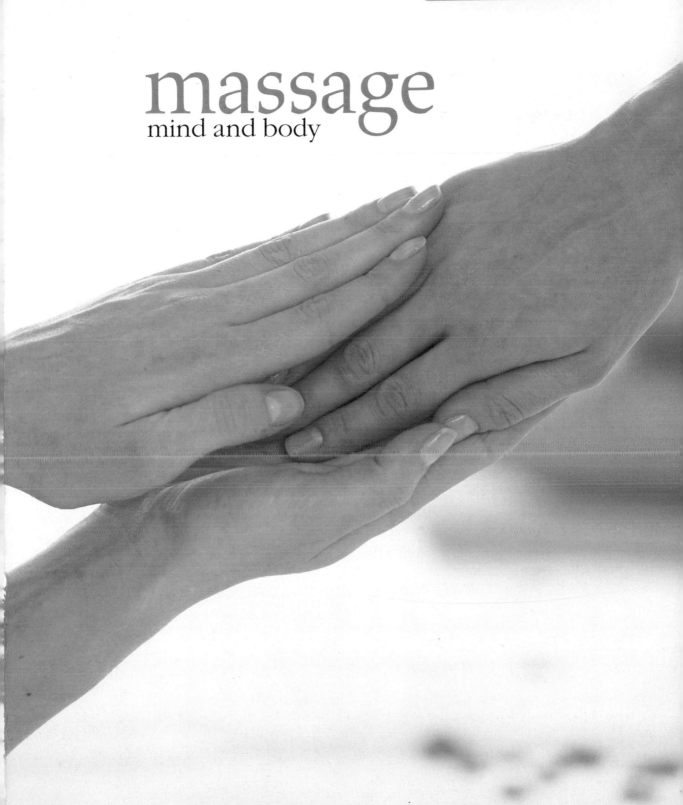

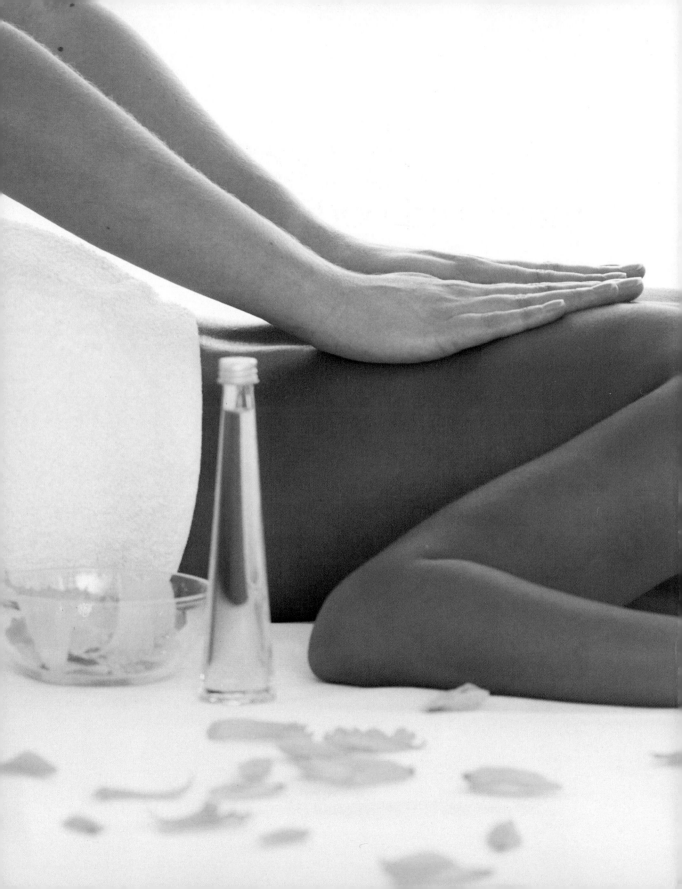

LARRY COSTA

massage
mind and body

PHOTOGRAPHY BY RUTH JENKINSON

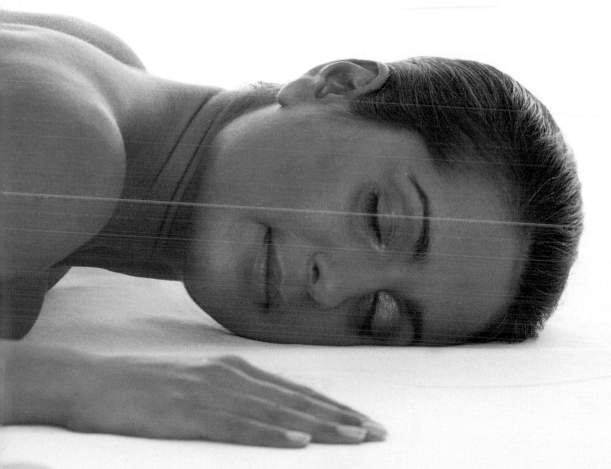

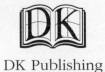

DK Publishing

LONDON, NEW YORK, MELBOURNE, MUNICH, and DELHI

For my family

Project Editor Nasim Mawji
Art Editor Miranda Harvey
Senior Editor Penny Warren
Senior Art Editor Sarah Rock
Managing Editor Stephanie Farrow
Category Publisher Mary-Clare Jerram
Art Director Carole Ash
DTP Designer Sonia Charbonnier
Production Controller Rita Sinha

Published in the United States by
DK Publishing, Inc.
375 Hudson Street
New York, New York 10014

First American edition, 2003
2 4 6 8 10 9 7 5 3 1

DK Publishing offers special discounts for bulk purchases for sales and promotions or
premiums. Specific, large-quantity needs can be met with special editions, including
personalized covers, excerpts of existing guides, and corporate imprints. For more
information, contact Special Markets Department, DK Publishing, Inc., 375 Hudson Street,
New York, New York 10014 Fax: 212-689-5254

Cataloging-in-Publication data for this book is available from the Library of Congress
ISBN 0-7894-9636-4

Color reproduction by Colourscan, Singapore
Printed and bound in Portugal by Printer Portuguesa

See our complete product line at
www.dk.com

CONTENTS

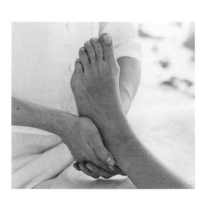
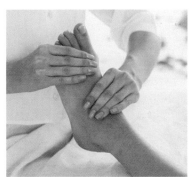
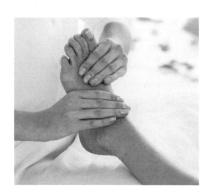

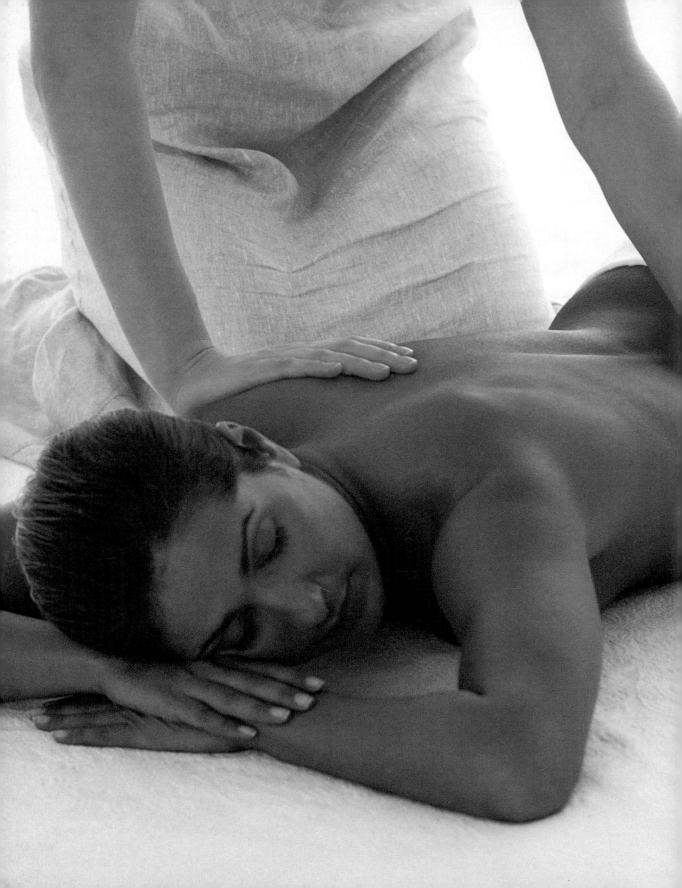

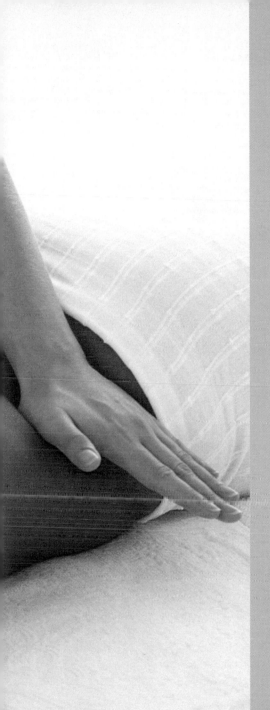

WHAT IS MASSAGE?

We've all appreciated a hug or a pat on the back—massage is just an extension of these forms of physical contact. This book teaches you how to use specific strokes and movements for the purpose of comforting, relaxing, easing pain, beautifying, soothing, and even offering emotional support. You'll find that it is as rewarding an experience to give a massage as it is to receive one.

DEFINING MASSAGE

From a very early age, our natural reaction when we hurt ourselves is to rub the injured area to soothe the pain. We are instinctively aware of the healing power of touch. Massage teaches us how to use touch for therapeutic benefit—to relax and soothe the body, and also the mind. With so many of today's health problems arising from stress, massage can have a profound and positive effect on our well-being.

Massage used to be considered an unnecessary luxury; today it is valued by many not only as one of the most effective means available for combating stress and inducing relaxation, but also for its many other physical and mental benefits, including expelling toxins, relieving muscle soreness, increasing flexibility, easing chronic pain, reducing tension headaches, boosting the immune system, promoting restful sleep, and improving concentration.

HOW MASSAGE WORKS

The human body is made up of different systems, among them the muscular, nervous, skeletal, lymphatic, cardiovascular, and digestive systems. Each system is affected, either directly or indirectly, by massage. After a massage you might expect your muscles to be relaxed, your senses to be heightened, your skeletal system to be realigned, your lymphatic system to be cleansed, your circulation to be improved, and your digestive system to function more smoothly. (Disorders such as constipation can be alleviated through massage.)

The first noticeable effect of massage on the body is a slight reddening of the skin in the area being worked on—this indicates that there is increased blood flow to that area. Improved circulation helps relieve many muscle ailments. When a muscle is tense and tight as a result of stress or injury, it contracts. This has the effect of squeezing some of the blood from the muscle, reducing circulation to it and causing the muscle fibers to cling together and become dry, like when cooked spaghetti is left to stand with no sauce. In severe cases, waste matter and toxins build up in the muscle fibers, and tense spots or "knots" develop, which feel like hard pebbles lodged deep within the muscle. If left untreated, the body begins to mistake these knots for bone and lays down calcium deposits on them. The results can be extremely painful.

When you massage a tense, contracted muscle, blood flow to it is increased, which helps to separate the muscle fibers. Think of this as putting sauce on spaghetti. The result is that toxins and waste matter are flushed from the cells and eliminated from the body through urination, defecation, and perspiration.

When one body system is adversely affected, other body systems are also impacted. Tense, contracted muscles affect the skeletal system by gradually pulling the bones out of alignment ultimately causing more pain and reducing mobility. Massage relaxes and can also help lengthen the muscles, which in turn realigns the skeleton. After a good massage, a person will often stand straighter and appear taller.

The physical benefits of massage are inextricably linked to an improved state of mind. Anxiety levels decrease, and people tend to sleep better after a massage. A well-rested person suffers less from exhaustion and fatigue and deals more effectively with stress. The ability to concentrate improves, and people tend to experience fewer tension headaches.

MUSCLE STRUCTURE

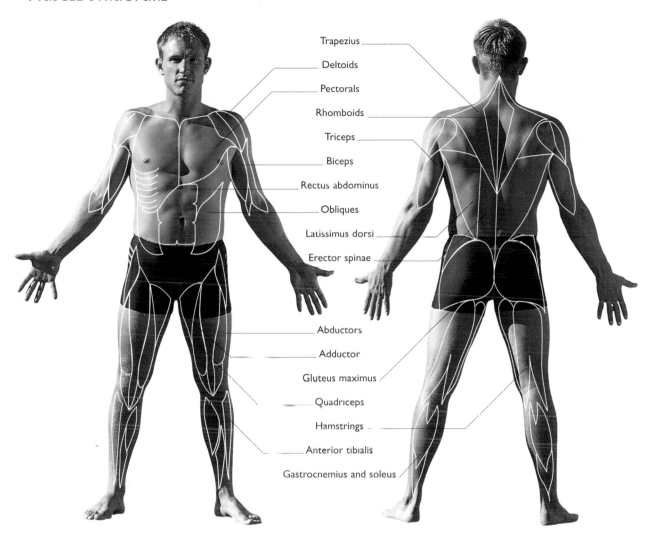

Trapezius
Deltoids
Pectorals
Rhomboids
Triceps
Biceps
Rectus abdominus
Obliques
Latissimus dorsi
Erector spinae
Abductors
Adductor
Gluteus maximus
Quadriceps
Hamstrings
Anterior tibialis
Gastrocnemius and soleus

At the front of the body weak abdominals can cause lower back pain; tense pectorals from lifting heavy weights cause shoulder pain; runners experience pain in the thighs.

At the back of the body tense neck muscles may cause headaches; people who drive long distances and women who wear heels may suffer from pains in the calves.

THE MUSCLES

Massage is manipulation of the body's muscle tissue, so to be a good masseur you need to be aware of how the different muscles are structured in the body. A massage stroke feels strangely incomplete if only part of the muscle is affected. You can learn a great deal about the health of the muscles—and the condition of the muscle fibers—simply by touching them. As your hands become more sensitive, you will notice that healthy muscle feels buoyant and offers less resistance, while tense muscle is harder and denser to the touch. With practice, you will also become more adept at sensing how the muscles respond to your touch.

PREPARING TO MASSAGE

All you really need to perform a massage is a pair of hands, but whether the aim is to soothe sore muscles or to ease tense ones, choosing a suitable oil or lotion helps to make the treatment more effective. Try using essential oils for their therapeutic qualities, and take time to create a relaxing environment by adjusting lighting and temperature and by making the person comfortable.

INGREDIENTS FOR MASSAGE

CARRIER OILS: My favorite oils for massage are sweet almond, grapeseed, and cold-pressed sunflower oils because they are light and easy to massage with, but you can also use wheatgerm and jojoba oils. If desired, essential oils may be added to any of these carrier oils. Olive oil is good for foot massages, and while you can use it on other parts of the body, avoid the face as it may clog pores. As a general rule, for a full body massage, you'll need about 4 tsp (20ml) of oil, for a back or neck and shoulder massage, about 1 tsp (5ml), and for a facial massage, use only a drop or two of oil.

LOTIONS: Ready-prepared massage lotions contain oils and tend to be greasy, so I prefer to make my own. Use any unscented, uncolored light lotion and either add an essential oil of your choice (*see chart*) or add a little oil to your palms, then rub a small amount of lotion into your hands before performing the massage. Lotion evaporates more quickly, so reapply it more often than when massaging with oil.

ESSENTIAL OILS: These highly concentrated plant extracts must be added to a carrier oil or unscented lotion. Do not apply them to the skin undiluted. Add 2–5 drops of essential oil to 2 tsp (10ml) of carrier oil or lotion.

NATURAL INGREDIENTS: Fresh fruit such as papayas, kiwis, pineapples, strawberries, bananas, and mangoes are great natural hydrators. They also contain enzymes that break down dead skin cells, exfoliating and rejuvenating the skin. A popular treatment at my spa consisted of a massage with puréed fresh winter melon, an Asian fruit that leaves the skin silky soft and nourished. For a fruit massage, use about three parts puréed fruit to one part oil. Fruit also makes an excellent ingredient for wraps. For natural exfoliators, experiment with grated fresh ginger, sea salt, oatmeal, poppy seeds, ground walnut shells, or even coarsely ground coffee mixed with just enough carrier oil to bind the ingredients.

Oil and lotion are popular choices for massage, or use ingredients such as puréed fruit and oatmeal—they nourish the skin and can also be used in wraps and as exfoliators.

CHOOSING ESSENTIAL OILS

The chart below lists my favorite essential oils along with their therapeutic properties. Be aware of the effects the different oils have before using them in a treatment. Keep essential oils away from eyes; never take them internally.

	essential oil	therapeutic property	caution
	Orange *Citrus aurantium*	Calming, sedative	May increase skin's sensitivity to sun
	Lemon *Citrus limonum*	Antibacterial, anti-inflammatory, calming	May increase skin's sensitivity to sun
	Eucalyptus *Eucalyptus globulus*	Antibacterial, soothes aches and pains, decongestant	
	Lavender *Lavandula angustifolia*	Anti-inflammatory, decongestant, calming, sedative, antidepressant	
	Peppermint *Mentha piperita*	Anti-inflammatory, decongestant, soothes aches and pains, energizing	Avoid in pregnancy
	Rose *Rosa x centifolia /* *Rosa x damascena*	Calming, uplifting, sedative	
	Rosemary *Rosmarinus officinalis*	Anti-inflammatory, decongestant, soothes aches and pains, uplifting	Avoid in pregnancy or if suffering from high blood pressure or epilepsy
	Clary sage *Salvia sclarea*	Antibacterial, decongestant, calming, antidepressant	Avoid in pregnancy

SETTING THE STAGE

A specially designed massage table is best for giving a massage, but at home you can improvise by using a futon or laying several blankets on the floor to create a firm but padded surface on which the person can lie. Beds, especially softer ones, are not ideal as they absorb the pressure of deeper strokes and can often be uncomfortable for the masseur.

When the person is lying on their front, place a rolled up towel or pillow under the ankles to prevent foot cramps and to relieve pressure on the knees when massaging the legs. Women may find a folded towel or pillow placed under the collar bone and chest comfortable. The best position for the arms is by the sides with palms facing up, but some people are more comfortable with arms raised by the head. It is fine for the person to adjust their position during the massage. When they are lying on their back, it can help relaxation to place a pillow under the knees to support them and prevent them from locking straight. You may also want to place a folded towel under the neck to help keep the body straight.

Body temperature drops during a massage so keep the room warm, slightly above normal room temperature. If the room is cold or drafty, the person will tense up. Cover areas not being worked on with a towel or blanket, and take care to keep the person's feet warm.

CREATING ATMOSPHERE

A massage can be given anywhere at any time, but you can make it special by taking a little time to prepare the room and to create some ambience.

Keep lights low, and avoid bright overhead lighting, which can be uncomfortable to look into when lying on the back. Candles provide a subtle and soothing light. Linens and sheets should be clean and unrumpled; otherwise they can be uncomfortable to lie on. Try laying down luxuriously textured fabrics such as velvets and silks or scattering a few fresh flower petals over the massage area. You may want to add a drop or two of essential oil to a diffuser, but be careful not to overdo it, and do not use chemical air fresheners—heavy scents are cloying and unpleasant.

Finally, any music should be soft and without lyrics; otherwise it can be distracting and intrusive. The atmosphere should be that of a peaceful and calming haven. The room should be free from chaos; all cares and worries are left at the door.

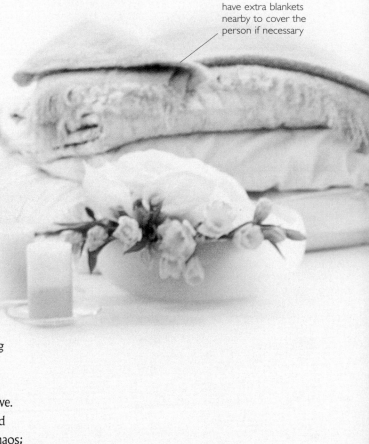

have extra blankets nearby to cover the person if necessary

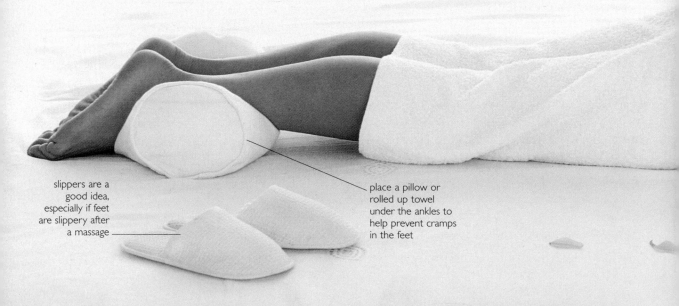

slippers are a good idea, especially if feet are slippery after a massage

place a pillow or rolled up towel under the ankles to help prevent cramps in the feet

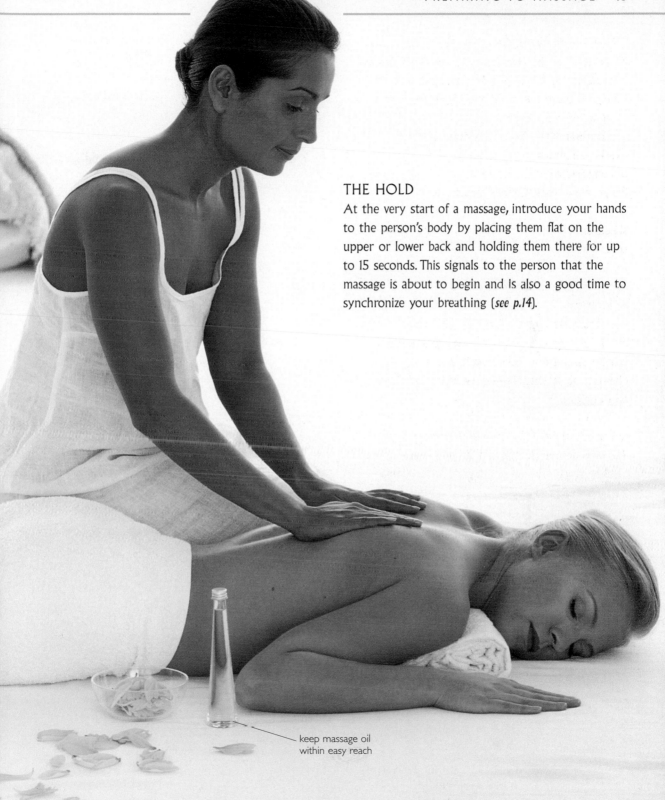

THE HOLD

At the very start of a massage, introduce your hands
to the person's body by placing them flat on the
upper or lower back and holding them there for up
to 15 seconds. This signals to the person that the
massage is about to begin and is also a good time to
synchronize your breathing (*see p.14*).

keep massage oil
within easy reach

APPLYING OIL

Pour a little oil into your palm rather than directly onto the body and rub your hands together to coat them and warm up the oil. Use enough oil to cover the area to be massaged with a light film. Your hands should glide easily over the skin, not create an oil slick.

BREATHING

Before you begin the massage, place your hands flat on the person's back and hold them there for several seconds. Ask the person to breathe in through the nose and out through the mouth as you do the same. Get a feel for the pace of the massage by sensing the rhythm of their breathing. Where possible, a good masseur tailors his strokes to move in time with the person's breathing—a stroke starts as the person inhales and is completed as he or she exhales.

PRESSURE

Begin a massage with gentle strokes to warm up the muscles to prepare them for deeper work and to stimulate blood flow to the area. The very act of touching has a therapeutic effect—there is no need to grab the muscle and wrestle it into submission. Start more tenderly and once the muscles are prepared, gradually increase the pressure. Watch the person's reaction: if you notice a grimace or a hand twitch, or if you feel a muscle tense up, ease up on the pressure.

As you learn how the muscles respond to your touch, it becomes easier to gauge the appropriate pressure. Throughout the treatments in this book I provide guidance on what pressure to use. It may vary from a light stroke, no more than a gentle brush against the skin, to firm pressure that requires you to put the weight of your body behind the movement.

MAINTAINING FLOW

Remember that each movement in a massage is seamlessly linked in a flowing sequence. Lifting your hands off the body is unsettling for the person being massaged and interrupts the flow. Maintain contact by keeping one hand on the body at all times, even when moving from one part of the body to another (*see below*). This allows the person to relax into the massage rather than anticipating your next move.

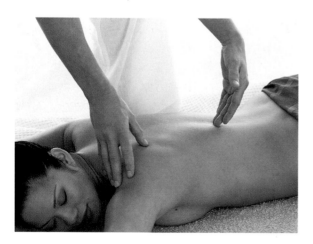

1 Moving from the shoulder to the side of the torso, the right hand maintains light contact with the shoulder as the left hand trails down the back.

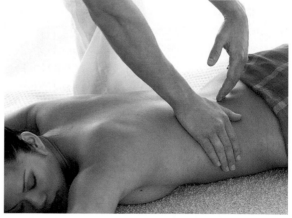

2 The right hand then glides down, meeting the left hand at the lower side of the torso to begin massaging that area.

HAND EXERCISES

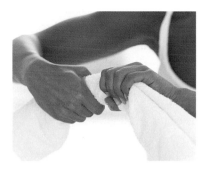

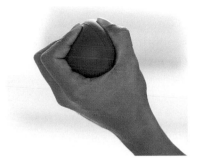

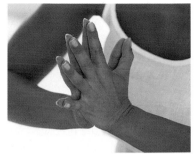

Towel twist Hold a rolled-up towel in front of you and practice wringing it, twisting it back and forth. Repeat 10 times. This strengthens the wrists and the forearms, areas prone to fatigue, especially during long or deep massages.

Ball squeeze Take a sponge ball or a squash ball, and practice squeezing it, then relaxing your hand. Squeeze 10 times with each hand. This strengthens the muscles in the palm, the back of the hand, and the fingers.

Finger stretch Hold your hands in front of you at chest height with fingers and palms touching. Lower your hands to stretch your wrists and fingers and stimulate blood flow to the wrists. Practice 10 times. This improves flexibility when massaging.

THE MASSEUR'S HANDS

Massage can be hard on your hands. You may find that your hands, wrists, and even your forearms tire easily, especially if performing long or particularly deep massages. Keeping your hands strong and flexible helps you to maintain regular rhythm when massaging. Strong hands allow you to exercise control when performing slow and fast strokes, and to maintain constant pressure. Hand exercises not only improve performance; they also help to prevent strain, fatigue, and even injury to the hands and wrists. Try the hand exercises above to help condition your hands for massage.

Always massage with clean hands, and take care to keep fingernails short or you may scratch. This is especially important when massaging delicate facial skin.

The hands, and sometimes the forearms, are used to massage, but don't be tempted to use other parts of the body. Avoid applying pressure with the knee or elbow, for example, as you won't be able to feel how the muscle responds; you are also very likely to cause pain and may even damage the tissue.

THE MASSEUR'S FRAME OF MIND

I believe that during a massage there is an exchange of energy between the masseur and the recipient. If you are tense, rushed, or distracted while giving a massage, the recipient will sense it in your hands and in your touch. Before you begin, use the breathing synchronization exercise (*see* Breathing *left*) to help you both to relax.

WHEN NOT TO MASSAGE

Avoid massaging directly on or in the area of broken skin or rashes, broken bones, or acute inflammation. Other unaffected areas of the body may still be massaged.

It is generally not advisable to massage a person with any of the following conditions: a high temperature, high blood pressure, a contagious disease, or cancer. Exercise extreme caution when massaging a woman in her first trimester of pregnancy: keep your strokes light and gentle, and avoid the lower back and abdomen.

POSTURES FOR MASSAGE

When you massage someone, you need to be able to move around and to adjust your position to reach different parts of the body and to perform each stroke effectively. For example, when massaging the back, kneeling by the side of the body helps your balance and also allows you plenty of control over pressure because you can lean your body weight into a stroke. Correct posture when massaging helps to prevent backache, minimize arm fatigue, and conserve your strength—while the person being massaged feels only a rhythmic and seamless flow of strokes.

KNEELING ON ONE KNEE

Use this position when performing long strokes where you need to reach to cover the whole area, for example, when massaging the leg. Control the pressure behind a stroke by shifting your body weight forward to increase intensity, and by sitting back on your heel to decrease it.

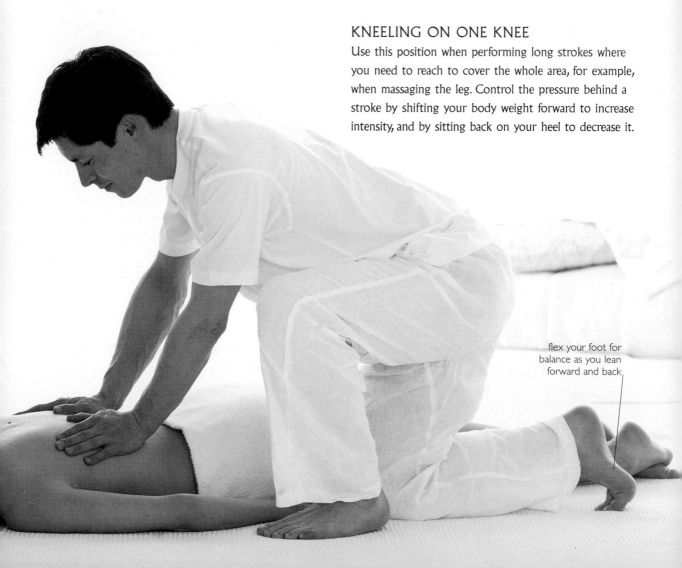

flex your foot for balance as you lean forward and back

KNEELING ON BOTH KNEES

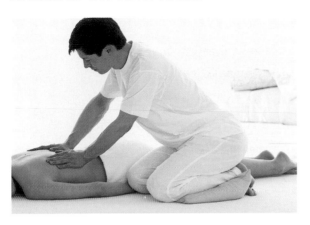

This is usually one of the most comfortable positions, especially with a small pillow or folded towel placed under the shins to relieve pressure on the knees and ankles. Sit back on the heels, or sit up and lean forward.

CROSS-LEGGED

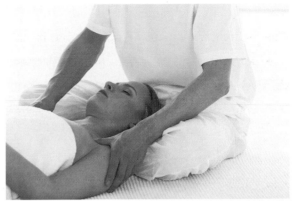

Sitting with your legs crossed creates a comfortable cradle for the head or the feet, and your calves will act as a cushion. Use this position for facials and head or foot massages where you are focusing on a single area.

SIDE-SADDLE

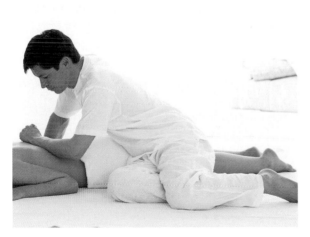

If performing a long massage on a single area, try sitting to the side of the person and leaning over them in the side-saddle position. Use this position for strokes that require little pressure. Try it too if you want to relieve pressure on your knees, ankles, and feet.

STRADDLE

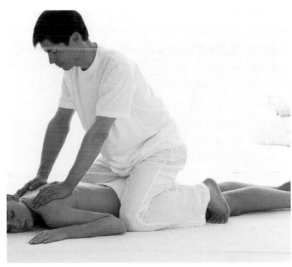

This maximizes physical contact between the person giving the massage and the recipient. Sit just below the person's bottom. This is a good position for back massage, but only straddle a person if you are both comfortable with it; it may be considered inappropriate.

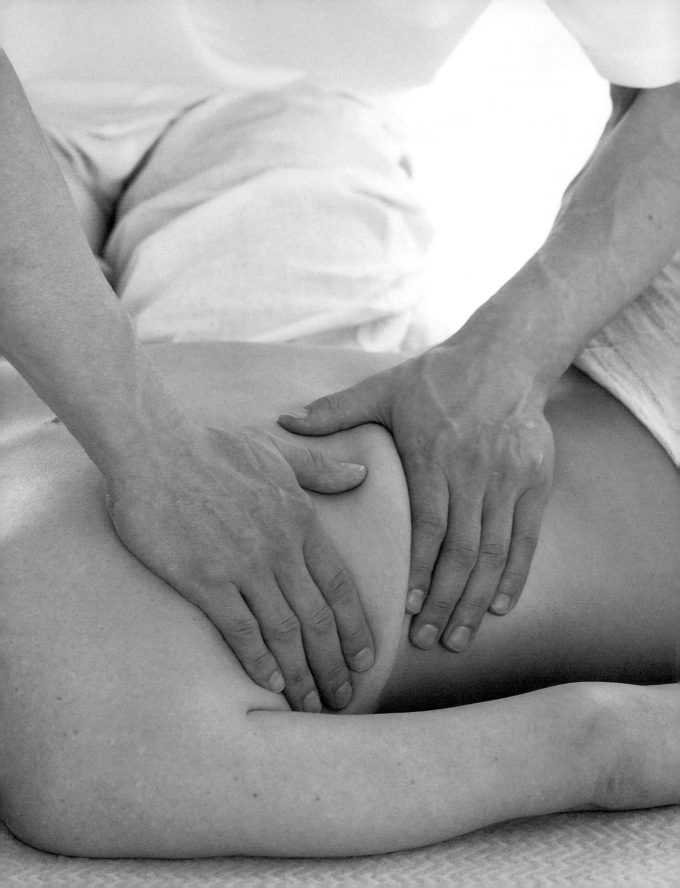

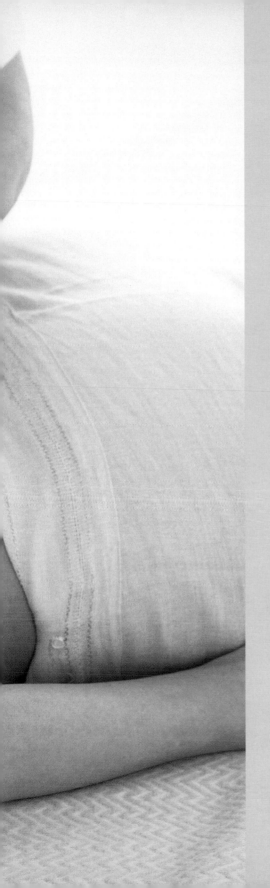

ESSENTIAL STROKES

The pages that follow will teach you the basic strokes and movements needed to perform a full body massage, as well as the many other routines and treatments in this book. These strokes provide you with a good grounding in basic massage technique, but there are many other strokes that are variations of these. As you become more confident, build up your repertoire by experimenting, adapting, and inventing new movements of your own.

STROKING

This is the most versatile massage technique: stroking gently and lightly has a calming and soothing effect, while increasing the pressure allows you to penetrate deeper into the muscles and stimulate blood flow to them. You could get away with mastering just this stroke and still give a perfectly good massage. Use stroking to slow the pace of a massage, for example when moving between brisk strokes. The key is to keep the movements smooth, rhythmic, and fluid.

APPLYING THE TECHNIQUE

• Use light long stroking at the start of a massage, then once the area is sufficiently relaxed, gradually increase the pressure.
• Synchronize the movement with the person's breathing when performing longer strokes on the back. Stroke as the person exhales.
• **Always** lighten the pressure when stroking over the backs of the knees.

keep fingers together and hands relaxed

ensure hands maintain full contact with the body

LIGHT LONG STROKING
best for back, legs, arms
Place your hands next to each other with fingers together. Glide your hands up the body, keeping the pressure light but constant. At the end of the stroke, slide your hands back to the start position and repeat.

STROKING WITH ALTERNATE HANDS
best for back, legs, arms
Position your hands as for light long stroking. Glide your right hand up the body, keeping your fingers together. Then glide your left hand up the body as your right hand slides back down to the start position. Repeat.

V-FORMATION STROKING best for back, abdomen, thighs

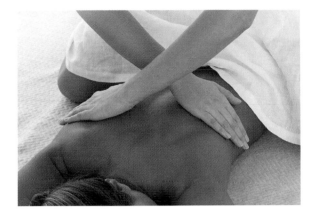

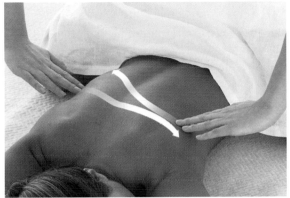

1 Place your left hand on the right side of the body and your right hand just below it on the left side, so that your wrists are crossed.

2 Slide your hands apart, then slide them in, moving your right hand up so that it finishes above your left. Both hands make V-shapes. Repeat the pattern, moving forward and alternating the leading hand.

HAND-OVER-HAND STROKING
best for back, legs, arms, torso

THUMB-OVER-THUMB STROKING
best for along spine, inside forearm, collar bone

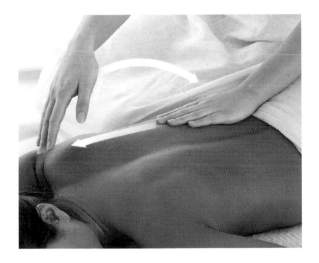

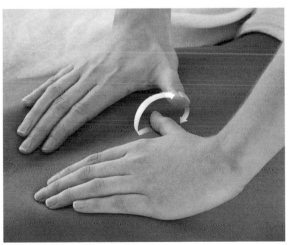

Place one hand on the lower back and gently glide it up the body. As you lift that hand off, begin gliding up the back with the other hand so that as one hand finishes a stroke, the other is about to begin (*see above*). You can also reverse the movement and stroke toward you, such as when reaching over the body to work on the side of the torso.

Place your hands next to each other on the body with fingers flat and thumbtips overlapping. Push forward with one thumb and, as you lift it off the body, push forward with the other thumb. Repeat, lifting one thumb over the other in a circular motion. When focusing work on smaller areas, it may be easier to lift your fingers off the body.

DEEP LONG STROKING
best for back, legs, arms

Begin in the same position as for light long stroking, with your hands next to each other on the body. Glide your hands forward, keeping your palms and fingers flat on the body and maintaining firm, constant pressure. As when light long stroking, maintain contact with the body by trailing your hands back to the starting position between strokes.

straighten arms and lean forward to increase pressure

HEEL-OF-HAND STROKING
best for back, thighs

Place the heel of your hand at the bottom of the area to be massaged, with fingers pointing upward. Press forward, following the direction of the muscle fibers. Put the weight of your body behind the movement, don't just press with your hand. This "irons out" the muscle, pressing it toward the bone and stimulating blood flow to it. Lift your hand off at the end of the stroke and repeat. The hand that is not massaging remains on the body to maintain contact. Use this stroke to concentrate pressure on particularly tight areas.

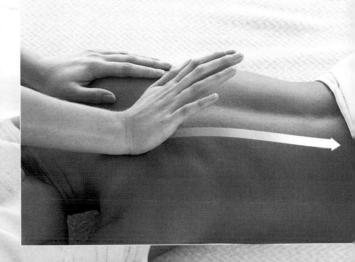

KNUCKLE STROKING
best for back, feet, thighs

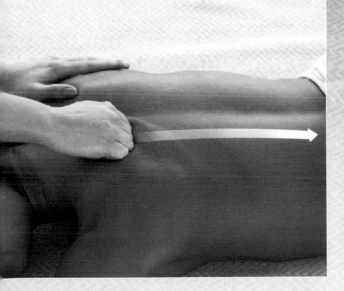

Make a loose fist and place it face down on the body. Glide your knuckles away from you, leaning into the stroke to apply firm, constant pressure. This penetrates deeper into the muscle than heel-of-hand stroking.

THUMB STRIPPING
best for back, forearms, shins

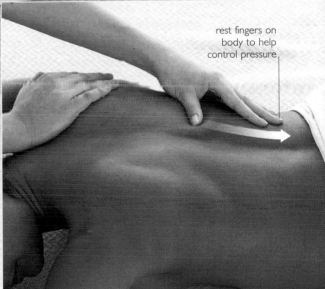

rest fingers on body to help control pressure

Place the side of your thumbtip against the body. Hold the skin taut with the other hand as you slide your thumb forward while applying firm pressure. This relaxes tense muscles by separating the muscle fibers.

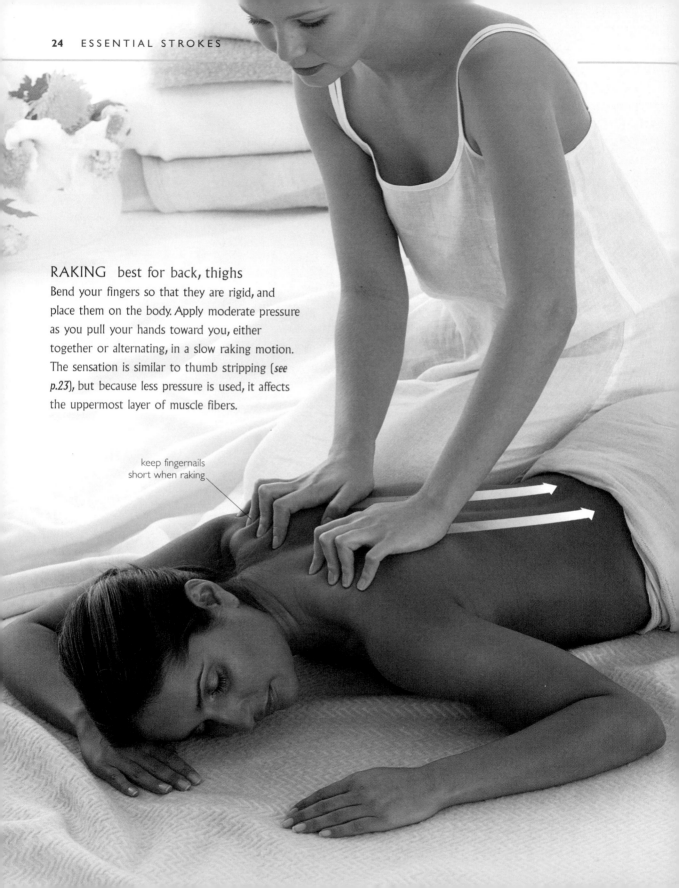

RAKING best for back, thighs

Bend your fingers so that they are rigid, and place them on the body. Apply moderate pressure as you pull your hands toward you, either together or alternating, in a slow raking motion. The sensation is similar to thumb stripping (*see p.23*), but because less pressure is used, it affects the uppermost layer of muscle fibers.

keep fingernails short when raking

DUSTING
best for entire body

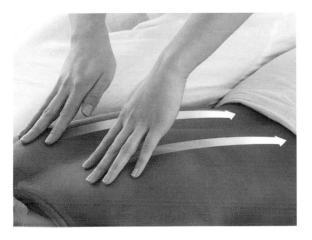

Very lightly stroke your fingertips toward you, either together or with alternate hands. This stroke gently stimulates the nerve endings under the skin and has a soothing, relaxing effect.

CROSS-FIBER WORK
best for along spine, shins, forearms

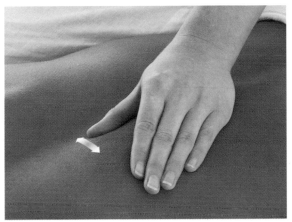

Place your hand on the body so that your thumb lies along the muscle fibers. With your thumb, make small movements back and forth across the muscle fibers, applying moderate pressure.

PAINTING   best for entire body

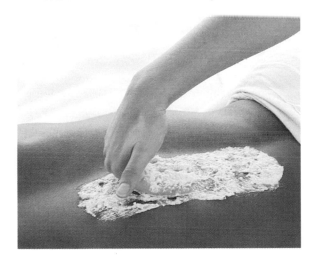

1 Apply exfoliant or wrap mixtures to the body with one hand and keep your free hand clean.

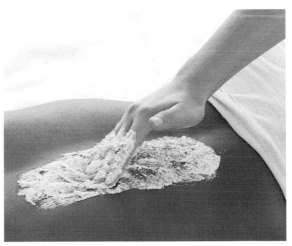

2 Use your fingers like a paintbrush, stroking them back and forth to spread the mixture.

FAN STROKING

This soothes and gently stimulates the nerve endings under the skin in the same way as light long stroking. Use variations of fan stroking to massage large areas—for example, try fanning your hands out at the end of the long stroke when massaging the back and legs. Use deeper strokes such as knuckle fanning to concentrate work on small areas. Where long stroking generally follows the direction of the muscle fibers, fan stroking provides a different sensation because the movement is across the muscles.

APPLYING THE TECHNIQUE
• Lighten the pressure on bony areas such as the upper back when performing forearm fanning.
• Apply confident pressure to the sides of the torso, the thighs, and the feet when performing finger fanning or knuckle fanning; these areas tend to be ticklish.

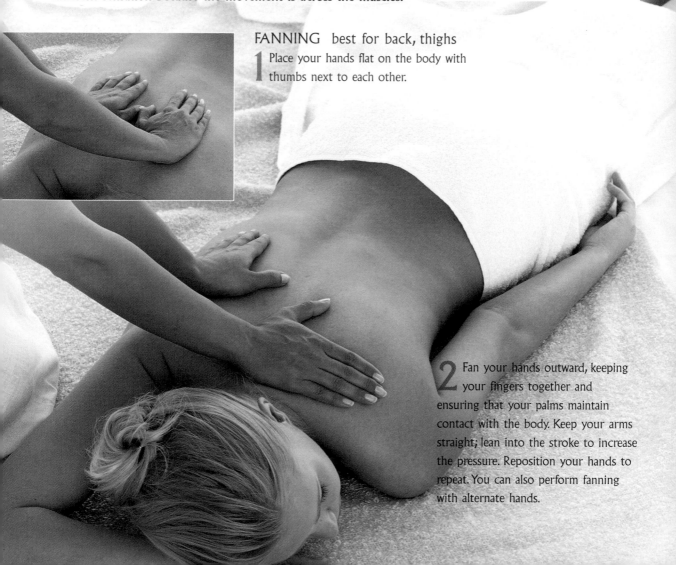

FANNING best for back, thighs

1 Place your hands flat on the body with thumbs next to each other.

2 Fan your hands outward, keeping your fingers together and ensuring that your palms maintain contact with the body. Keep your arms straight; lean into the stroke to increase the pressure. Reposition your hands to repeat. You can also perform fanning with alternate hands.

FOREARM FANNING best for back, thighs

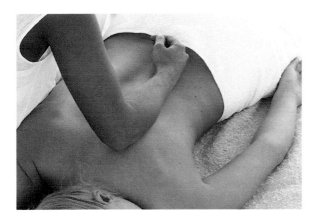
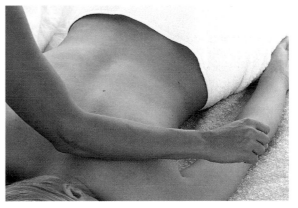

1 Bend your elbow, make a loose fist, and place the fleshiest part of your forearm (not the sharp bone at the front of the arm) against the body.

2 Turn your wrist inward slightly to maximize muscle-to-muscle contact and, with your arm, stroke away from you, pivoting from your elbow.

FINGER FANNING
best for lower back, thighs

KNUCKLE FANNING
best for lower back, feet, buttocks, neck, face

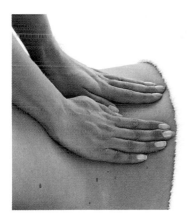
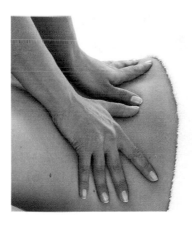
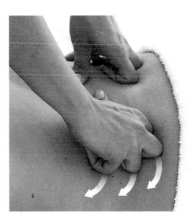

1 Place your hands next to each other, flat against the body with thumbs touching.

2 Leading with your little finger, fan outward applying pressure with each finger as you fan.

Curl your fingers under your hand, and fan out with your knuckles, leading with your little finger.

KNEADING

Although kneading is one of the most popular massage strokes, it is almost always performed incorrectly. For both kneading and lifting, the aim is to compress the muscle gently, stimulating blood supply to it and providing it with oxygen and nutrients that can soothe soreness and also help rebuild damaged tissue. Be firm and confident as you grasp the flesh, and take care not to pinch the skin because this will be painful. You may vary the pace, but keep your movements rhythmic.

APPLYING THE TECHNIQUE

• Keep your fingers together when performing the kneading and lifting strokes—splayed fingers will tickle and cause the person to tense up.
• Don't worry if skin reddens slightly; this indicates increased blood flow.
• **Avoid** kneading or lifting directly over varicose veins. Skim over them to the next area, or massage next to them.

keep fingers together

grasp flesh firmly

TWO-HANDED KNEADING best for fleshy areas

1 Kneel at one side of the body, and reach over to knead the side furthest from you. Place both hands flat on the body with elbows out to the sides, and take a firm hold of a good handful of flesh with your left hand.

ONE-HANDED KNEADING best for fleshy areas, legs, arms

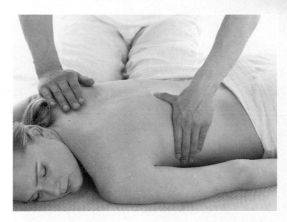

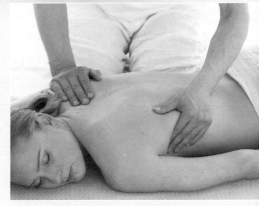

1 Make a wide V-shape with your thumb and index finger, and place your hand flat against the body with fingers together. Rest your other hand nearby on the body to maintain contact.

2 Grasp the flesh and push it forward and upward, firmly pressing your hand against the body. Keep your fingers straight and together.

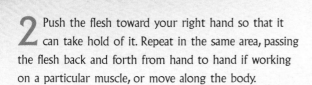

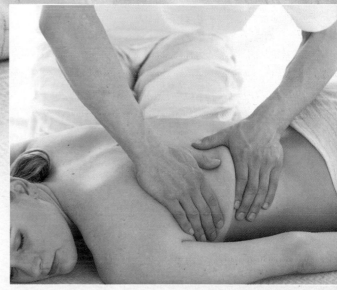

2 Push the flesh toward your right hand so that it can take hold of it. Repeat in the same area, passing the flesh back and forth from hand to hand if working on a particular muscle, or move along the body.

FINGERTIP KNEADING best for fleshy areas, lower back, feet, hands

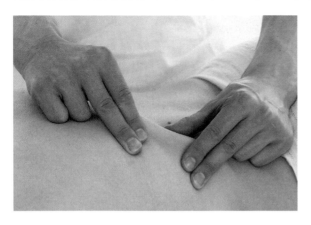 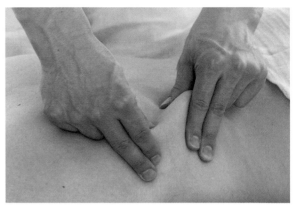

1 Lift a small fold of flesh between the first two fingers and thumb of your right hand and gently pull upward. If you rest your hands lightly on the body, you can control the pressure as you knead.

2 Gently push the flesh toward your left hand, then release it so the fingers and thumb of your left hand can take hold of it. Repeat, passing the flesh from one hand to the other.

THUMB KNEADING best for forearms, lower back

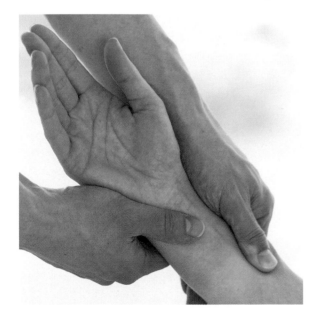 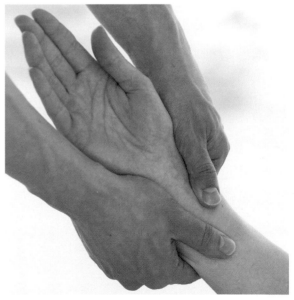

1 Place your right thumb at the base of the forearm and your left a little higher up. Using the pad and side of your left thumb, push the flesh upward and outward.

2 Move your right hand up the arm. Repeat the action with the right thumb, pushing the flesh upward and outward as you move up the forearm.

LIFTING best for calves, biceps

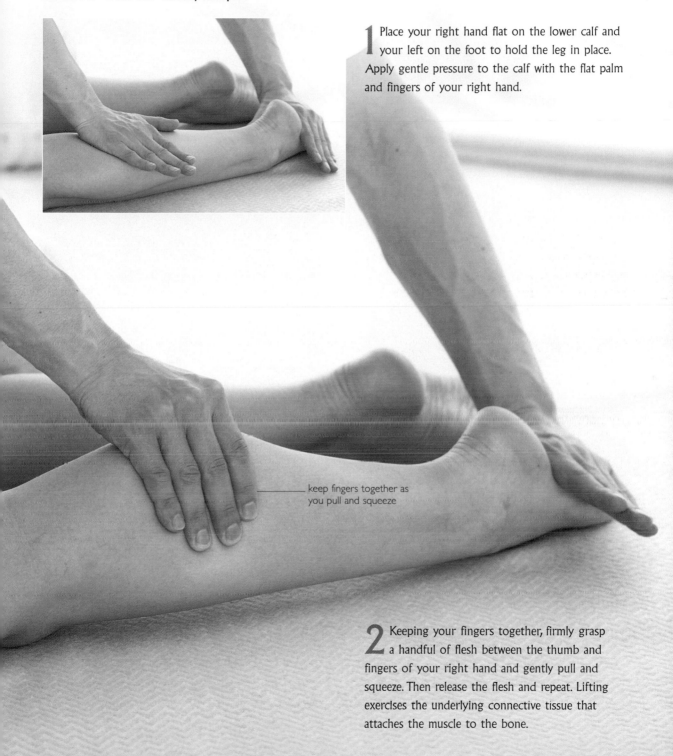

1 Place your right hand flat on the lower calf and your left on the foot to hold the leg in place. Apply gentle pressure to the calf with the flat palm and fingers of your right hand.

keep fingers together as you pull and squeeze

2 Keeping your fingers together, firmly grasp a handful of flesh between the thumb and fingers of your right hand and gently pull and squeeze. Then release the flesh and repeat. Lifting exercises the underlying connective tissue that attaches the muscle to the bone.

PRESSURES

Pressure may be concentrated in a small area, such as when using finger pressure to stimulate an acupressure point. Or you can use techniques to apply slightly greater pressure to broader areas, such as the lower back or the arms or legs, where the effect will be to stretch and compress the muscle, stimulating blood flow to it. When increasing the pressure during a movement or stroke, always ask the person for feedback. You may apply very firm pressure in some cases, but you should never cause pain.

APPLYING THE TECHNIQUE
• Use enough oil or lotion for your hands to glide when performing strokes that combine pressure with movement, such as heel-of-hand compressions (*opposite*) and corkscrew thumb pressure (*p.35*); avoid pulling or stretching the skin.
• **Be sure** to locate acupressure points accurately before applying gradually increasing pressure.

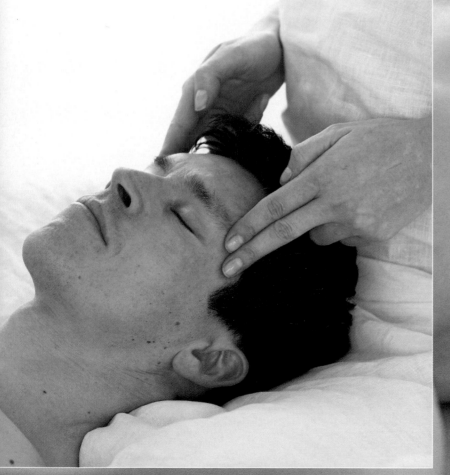

FINGER PRESSURE
best for acupressure points, entire body
With one or more fingers, apply gradually increasing pressure, hold for 3–4 seconds, then gently release. You can also massage with circular movements. Finger pressure is most commonly used on the temples or the base of the skull when treating stress headaches. To apply less pressure, use your middle or ring finger.

HEEL-OF-HAND COMPRESSION
best for back, legs, arms, neck, shoulders

Place the heels of your hands against the body.
Keeping your fingers up and away from the body,
lean forward and straighten your arms to
increase the pressure. Hold for 3–4
seconds, then slowly release.

raise fingers to
concentrate
pressure on
heels of hands

FULL-HAND COMPRESSION best for back, arms, legs

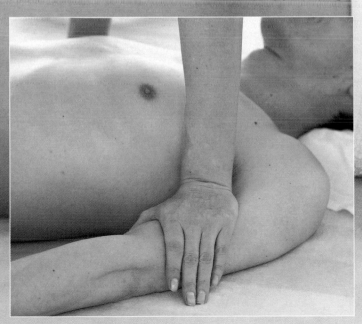

Place your hand on the
body, ensuring that your
fingers and palm are in
contact with it. Apply
pressure by leaning into
the movement for 3–4
seconds, then ease off
for 3–4 seconds. When
performing this over
a large area, try to
keep pressure even
from the heel of the
hand to the fingertips.

KNUCKLE PRESSURE best for upper back, thighs, calves

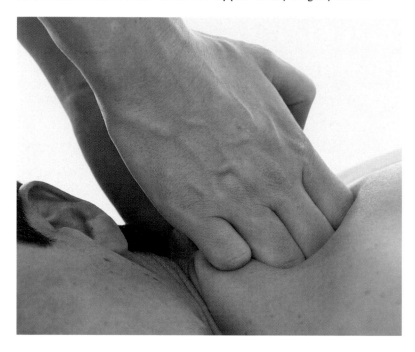

Curl your fingers under your hands and place them against the body, concentrating pressure on the knuckles of your middle fingers. Apply gradually increasing pressure, hold for 3–4 seconds, then gently release. To increase the pressure, lean into your middle knuckles, putting your body weight behind them and keeping your arms straight.

THUMB PRESSURE best for acupressure points, entire body

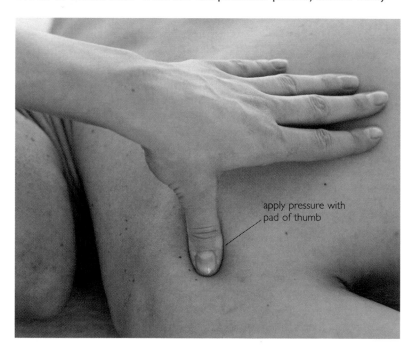

apply pressure with pad of thumb

Press with your thumb to stimulate pressure points or to break up stress knots that tend to occur in the neck and shoulder area, back, and feet. Apply gradually increasing pressure, hold for 3–4 seconds, then slowly release. Rest your hand on the body to help control pressure.

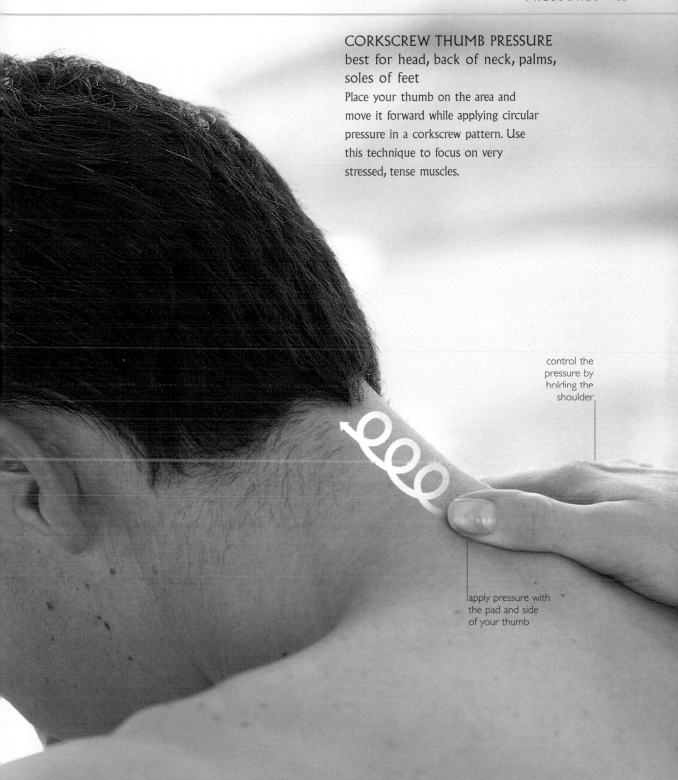

CORKSCREW THUMB PRESSURE
best for head, back of neck, palms, soles of feet
Place your thumb on the area and move it forward while applying circular pressure in a corkscrew pattern. Use this technique to focus on very stressed, tense muscles.

control the pressure by holding the shoulder

apply pressure with the pad and side of your thumb

PERCUSSION

Gentle tapping with the fingertips, pummeling with the fists, or hacking with the sides of the hands all stimulate the nerve endings under the skin and have an exhilarating effect. Along with tweaking, cupping, and slapping, these strokes can help to tone muscles and also increase circulation. Use these strokes when you have finished massaging an area or at the end of a massage session. Generally, percussion strokes are better for fleshy areas, and more bony areas of the body should be avoided.

APPLYING THE TECHNIQUE
• Keep wrists loose and relaxed when performing any percussion strokes.
• Relax a tense muscle with gentler strokes before progressing to hacking or pummeling.
• Keep hands cupped when performing cupping, and listen for a hollow sound.
• **Never** perform pummeling or hacking over the spine or kidney area.

FINGER TAPPING best for entire body

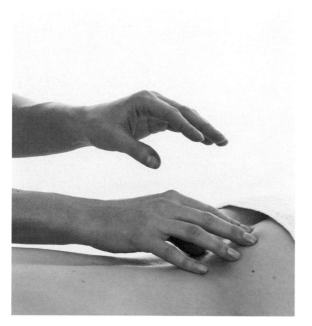

Use the pads of your fingertips in a gentle tapping action. Tap all fingers simultaneously or drum your fingers to create a gentle vibration that stimulates nerve endings and promotes circulation. This stroke is commonly used in facial massage for its invigorating and toning effects.

PUMMELING best for lower back, buttocks

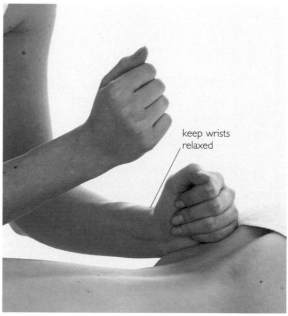

keep wrists relaxed

This technique is performed with relaxed wrists and loosely formed fists. Each stroke should bounce off the body. Pummel simultaneously or with alternate hands, either directly on the body or through a towel. Rhythmic pummeling sends resonating vibrations through an area so the entire muscle is affected.

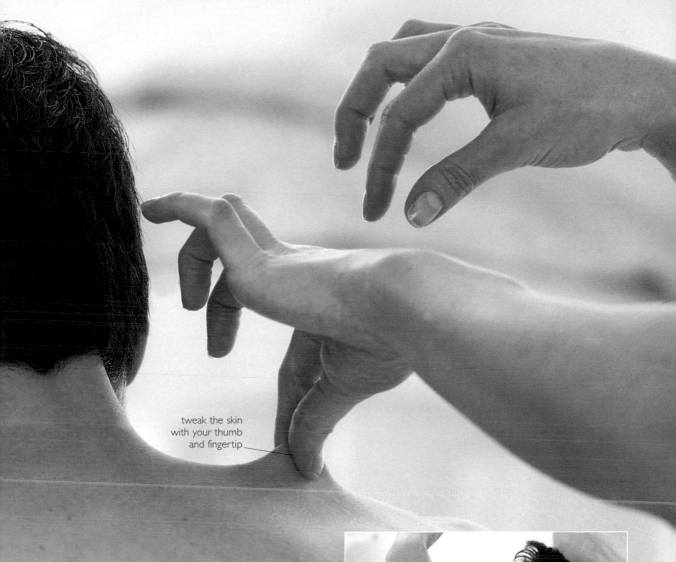

tweak the skin
with your thumb
and fingertip

TWEAKING best for shoulders, face, toes
Gently pick up some skin between your thumb and
index finger, taking care not to pinch, then release it.
Repeat with alternate hands, maintaining a fast-paced,
steady rhythm. Use tweaking on tense, stressed muscles
anywhere in the body.

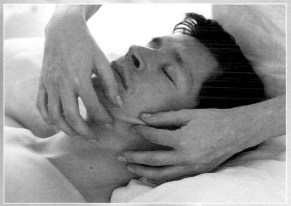

Very gentle but brisk, rhythmic tweaking on the face,
especially along the jaw line, can help tone slack skin
and jowls. Take care not to tug the skin.

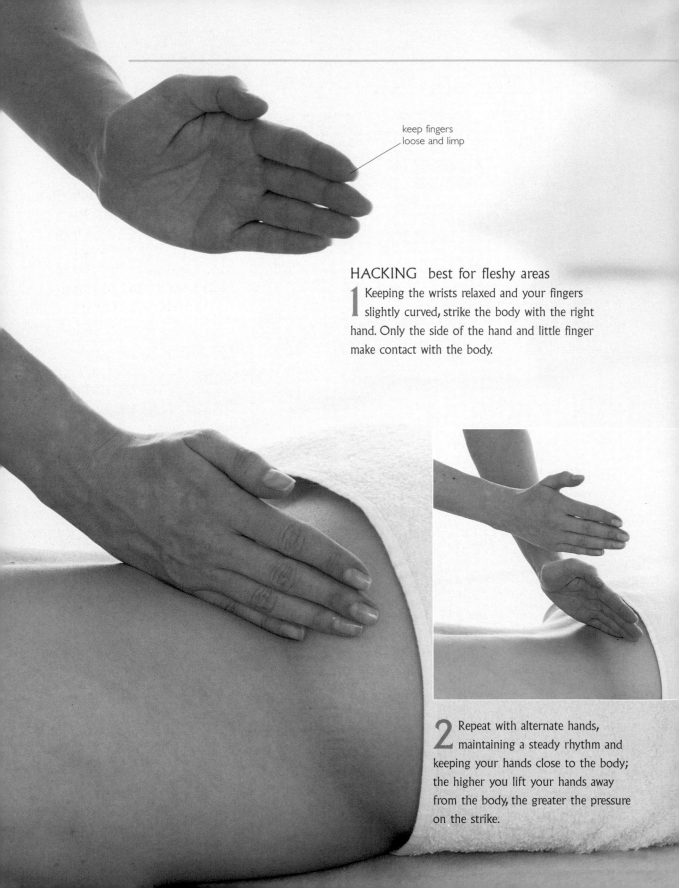

keep fingers
loose and limp

HACKING best for fleshy areas

1 Keeping the wrists relaxed and your fingers slightly curved, strike the body with the right hand. Only the side of the hand and little finger make contact with the body.

2 Repeat with alternate hands, maintaining a steady rhythm and keeping your hands close to the body; the higher you lift your hands away from the body, the greater the pressure on the strike.

CUPPING best for thighs, buttocks, upper arms

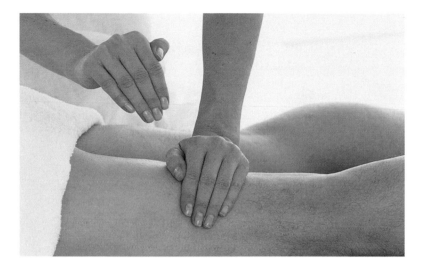

Cup your hands with slightly bent fingers as if holding water. Tap the area with alternate hands or simultaneously. As you place your cupped hand on the body, air is trapped under it, then suction is created as you lift your hand away. This has the effect of stimulating blood flow closer to the surface of the skin, which helps to oxygenate the muscles and eliminate toxins.

SLAPPING best for face, entire body

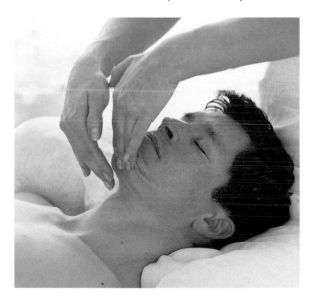

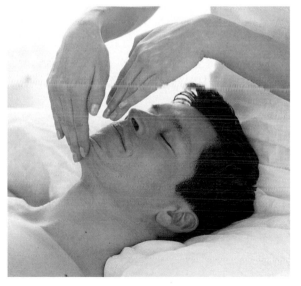

1 Sweep your fingertips up the chin, keeping your wrist relaxed and your fingers together. Use light pressure, especially when working on the face.

2 Repeat the stroke using alternate hands, working along the jaw line. This stimulates the nerve endings under the skin, promoting pleasant sensations of tingling and warmth.

FRICTION

Use a technique such as brisk sawing to stimulate the nerve endings on the surface of the skin and to warm up tired, sore, or achy muscles at the start of a massage. Techniques such as cross-fiber friction and twisting penetrate deeper into the muscle fibers, increasing blood flow to the muscles and helping to flush away toxins—use these strokes only when the muscles have been sufficiently warmed up. Friction strokes can follow the direction of the muscle fibers or be performed across them.

APPLYING THE TECHNIQUE

• Notice that skin reddens slightly when performing repetitive friction strokes in one area; this indicates an increase in blood flow and causes a pleasant tingling sensation.

• **Take care** not to overdo it. If working in one area, move slightly to the side, then work back to that area to avoid causing an unpleasant burning sensation.

SAWING   best for back, feet, fleshy areas

1 Place your hands about 1–2in (2–4cm) apart on the body with palms facing. Keep your fingers and wrists relaxed.

2 Briskly rub the sides of your hands back and forth on the body with a sawing motion. This is the fastest of all the strokes. You should notice a slight reddening of the skin. Take care not to jab with your fingertips as you saw.

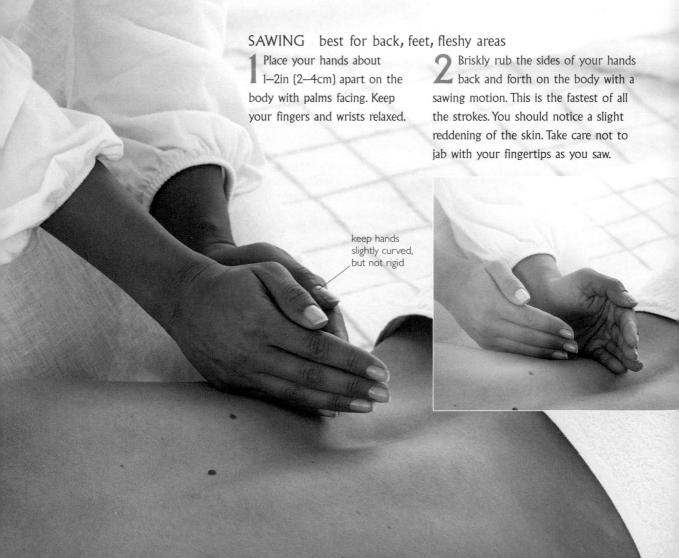

keep hands slightly curved, but not rigid

CROSS-FIBER FRICTION best for hands, feet

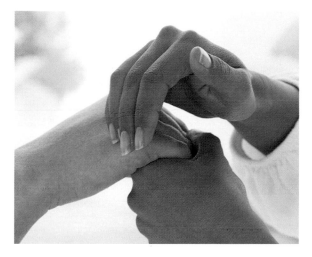

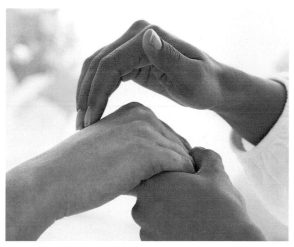

1 Hold the person's hand with one hand and, cupping your hand slightly, sweep the pads of your fingertips across the top of the hand. Keep your wrists and fingers relaxed.

2 Repeat the action, sweeping your fingers briskly back and forth across the top of the hand. This movement affects the underlying muscles and tendons, separating the muscle fibers and increasing blood flow.

TWISTING best for fingers, toes

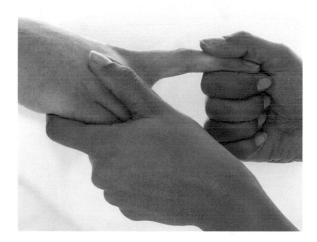

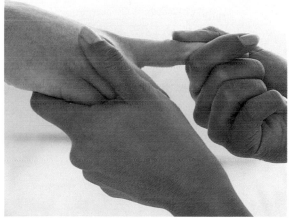

1 Curl your fingers into your palm and grasp the person's finger between your thumb and the knuckle of your index finger. Apply gentle but firm pressure with your thumb.

2 Gently twist the skin in one direction and then in the other, working each section of the finger and then the thumb individually. This compresses the muscles against the bones, stimulating blood flow to the muscles.

VIBRATION

This can be anything from a gentle rocking of the entire body to a tremulous shaking motion concentrated on a single area. Try combining vibration with strokes such as the long stroke, and experimenting with the technique by varying the pace and the pressure of the vibration. If performed slowly and rhythmically with very light pressure, the stroke is soothing, relaxing, and positively tension-diffusing. Applied with greater pressure, vibration can be invigorating and also helps to release toxins from the muscles.

APPLYING THE TECHNIQUE
• Don't let the person help you when performing any of these strokes. Sometimes people will try to rock their body for you or help you by lifting their arm. Encourage the person to relax.
• **Avoid** performing the stroking with vibration technique (*p.45*) before other tiring strokes such as kneading. Use this stroke to finish work on a body part.

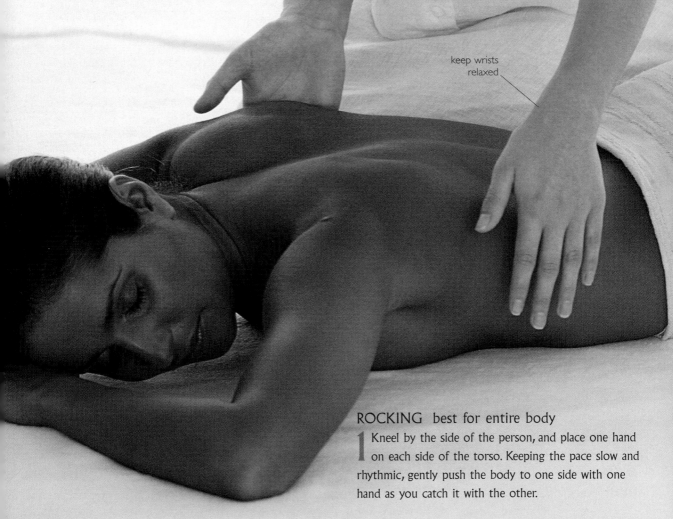

keep wrists relaxed

ROCKING best for entire body
1 Kneel by the side of the person, and place one hand on each side of the torso. Keeping the pace slow and rhythmic, gently push the body to one side with one hand as you catch it with the other.

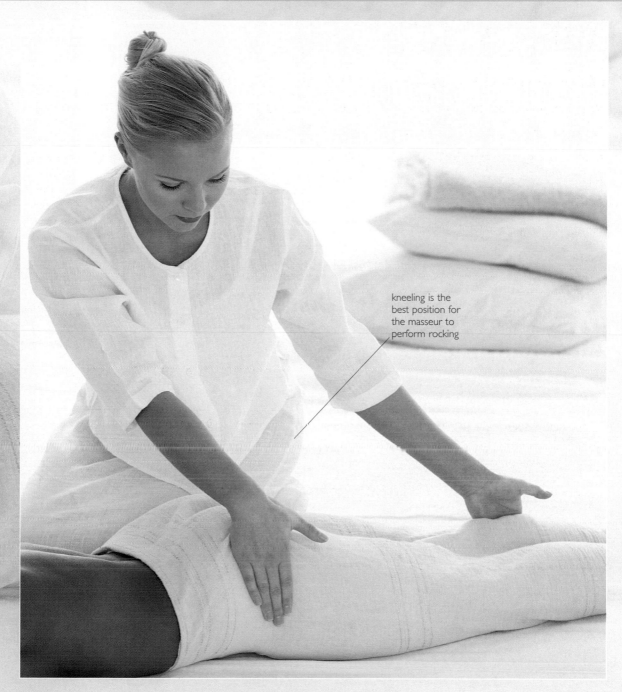

kneeling is the
best position for
the masseur to
perform rocking

2 Move further down the body, placing one hand on the hip
and the other lower down on the leg. Continue to rock the
body gently, pushing it from one hand to the other. As the person
relaxes, you'll notice that it takes less effort to rock the body.

ROLLING best for arms, lower legs

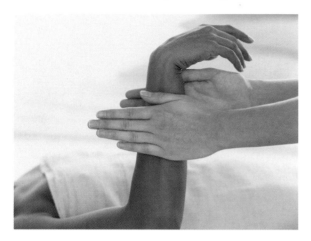

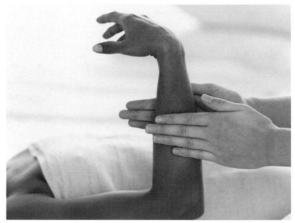

1 Hold the relaxed limb between your palms, taking care to keep your fingers straight and together. Start with one hand positioned a little higher than the other.

2 Apply gentle pressure to compress the muscle against the bone as you gently roll the limb back and forth between your hands.

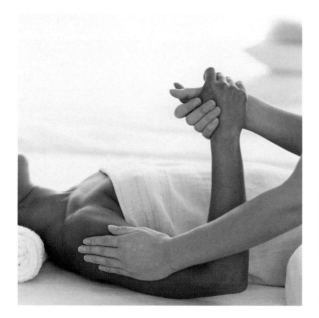

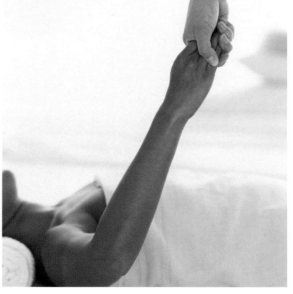

SHAKING best for entire body
Use this technique to locate areas of tension in the body. Place your hand over the area and, applying light pressure, gently shake it. If the body part does not vibrate and move loosely under your hand, there is tension.

SWINGING best for arms, legs
Use this technique to relax the limbs. Take hold of the the person's limb and lift it up. If the arm feels light, it is not relaxed. Gently swing the arm back and forth, noticing that it feels heavier as it relaxes.

STROKING WITH VIBRATION
best for entire body

Combine vibration with the long stroke. Place your hand flat against the body and, as you stroke, apply gentle pressure combined with shaking. Use gentle pressure for a soothing effect, and increase the pressure and the pace of the vibration for a more invigorating effect. Use your whole arm, not just your wrist, to generate the vibration.

keep fingers together and hand flat against body

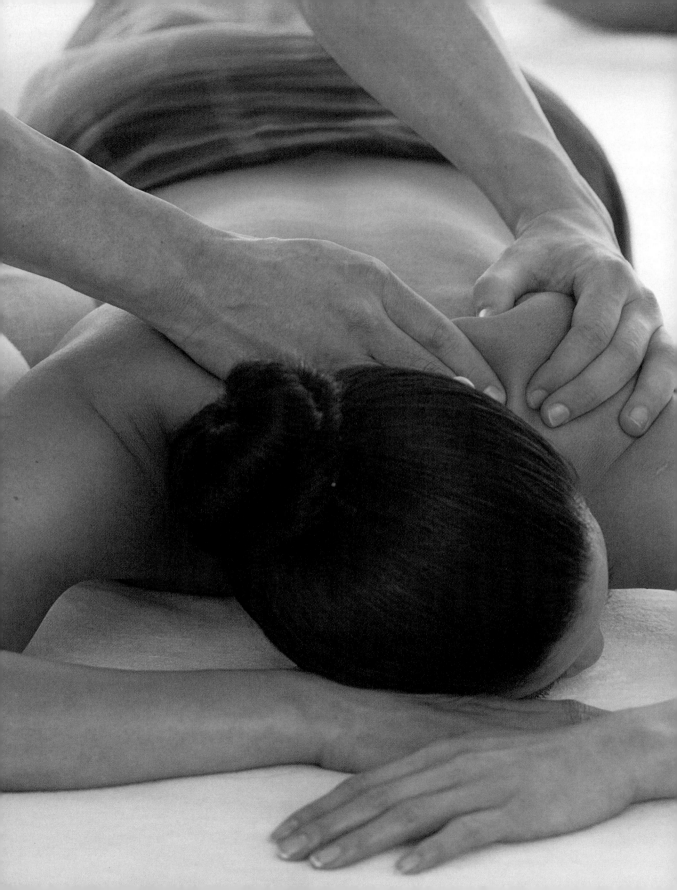

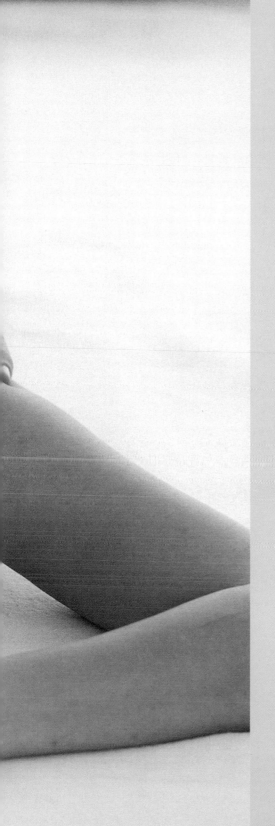

FULL BODY MASSAGE

This is an adapted version of my famous full body massage. Here I guide you through a soothing massage that flows from one part of the body to the next. Follow the routine from start to finish, or use part of it to work on a particular area of the body. The massage takes about an hour, but you could easily take longer. Spend more time on tense muscles or just on areas that the person enjoys having massaged. Use oil or lotion (see *pp.10–11*).

THE BACK

A good back massage is one of life's most profoundly relaxing experiences. It can be so effective at relieving stress that I have even had people cry with relief as I ease out knots and muscle tension with a combination of rhythmic strokes and carefully applied pressure. Take care to lighten the pressure and to avoid any percussion strokes when massaging in the kidney area (in the small of the back).

1 Kneel at the person's head, and place the heels of your hands at the base of the lower back. Perform a HEEL-OF-HAND COMPRESSION by leaning forward with straight arms and applying firm pressure for 10 seconds, then releasing.

raise fingers to concentrate pressure on heels of hands

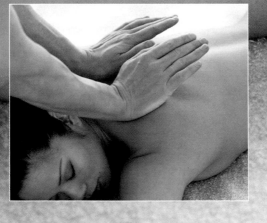

2 Then walk your hands up the back performing HEEL-OF-HAND COMPRESSIONS with alternate hands. Be sure to avoid the kidney area. At the shoulders, slide back down to the buttocks and work up the back again. Repeat at least 3 times, finishing on the upper back.

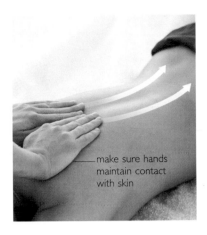

make sure hands maintain contact with skin

3 Perform LIGHT LONG STROKING down the back 3 times. Keep your fingers together as you stroke. At the end of the third stroke down, leave your hands in position on the lower back.

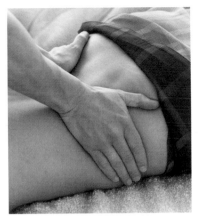

4 Perform FANNING, working up the back to the shoulders 3 times. This elongates the muscles on the sides of the torso as well as along the back. Leave one hand on the body to maintain contact as you move around to the person's side.

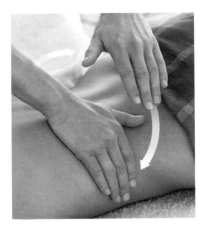

5 Lean over to perform HAND-OVER-HAND STROKING, pulling the skin toward you as you apply moderate pressure. Work up to the arm and down again 3 times. Then move your hands to the shoulders, ready to perform kneading.

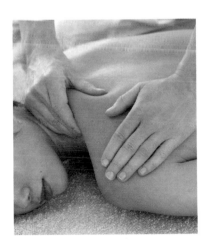

6 Perform TWO-HANDED KNEADING to the shoulders. Grasp and gently squeeze the flesh with one hand, then pass it to the other to do the same. Begin kneading more firmly and continue, maintaining a rhythm, until the muscle relaxes.

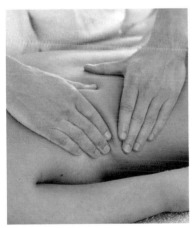

7 Ease the pressure slightly as you move to the side of the body to continue TWO-HANDED KNEADING. Work this area intensively, moving up and down the side for at least a minute and establishing a rhythm as you knead.

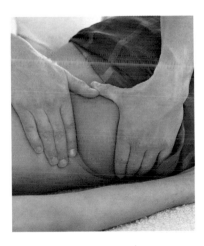

8 Move down to the lower side of the body and, maintaining your rhythm, perform TWO-HANDED KNEADING to the fleshy area there. Then, maintaining contact with the body, slide your hand to the top of the back to begin thumb stripping.

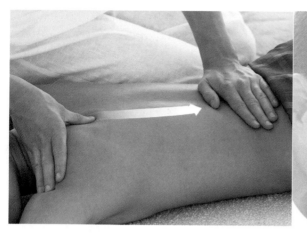

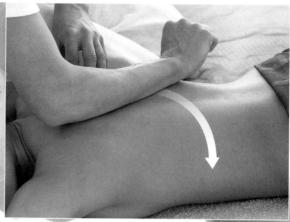

9 Place your left hand on the lower back and, with your right hand, perform THUMB STRIPPING along the muscles on the side of the spine furthest from you. Repeat several times, sliding your thumb slowly over the muscles and maintaining firm, constant pressure.

10 Bend your elbow and turn your wrist inward. Place the fleshy part of your forearm against the back and perform FOREARM FANNING to the side furthest from you. Repeat 4–6 times, moving down the back, applying moderate pressure to "iron out" the muscles.

11 Then begin FOREARM-OVER-FOREARM STROKING. Lean forward to increase the pressure, and try to maintain a steady rhythm. Repeat several times, concentrating on the side of the back closest to you.

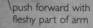
push forward with fleshy part of arm

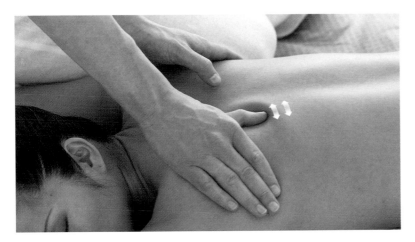

12 Position your hand at the top of the back to begin CROSS-FIBER WORK on the muscles along the side of the spine furthest from you. Rest your hand on the back to help control the pressure you apply with your thumb. Work down the back at least 3 times. Finish with your hand on the lower back.

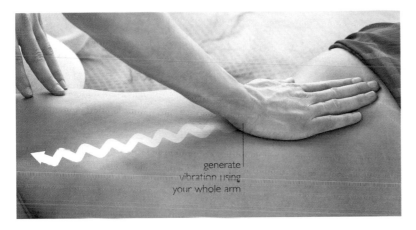

generate vibration using your whole arm

13 Perform STROKING WITH VIBRATION, working up the spine from the lower back to the shoulders. Ensure that your entire hand maintains contact with the body. Vibrate the skin gently, leaning forward to increase the pressure. Repeat, working up first one side of the spine and then the other.

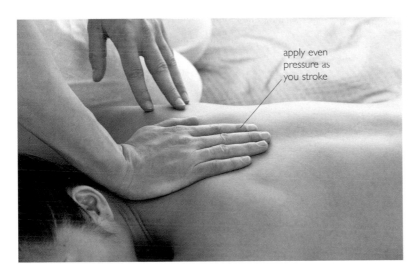

apply even pressure as you stroke

14 Perform LIGHT LONG STROKING over the entire back. Then move around and sit to the other side of the person. Repeat steps 5–14 on the other side of the back. End the back massage here or, if you are giving a full body massage, move to the feet to start massaging the legs.

THE LEGS

Don't be afraid to use firm pressure when massaging the meaty muscles in the legs, but do be careful to lighten the pressure when stroking over the back of the knee, and never massage directly over this area or on the kneecap. You may want to place a rolled-up towel or a small cushion under the person's ankles when lying on the front, since this can help to prevent foot cramps.

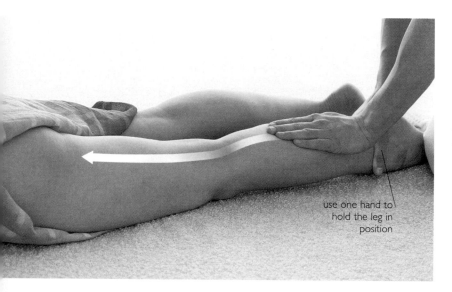

use one hand to hold the leg in position

1 With the person lying on his or her front, begin with the left leg. Kneel by the left foot and hold the leg by the ankle with your right hand. Keeping your left hand flat and your fingers together, stroke up to the top of the leg. Lighten the pressure over the back of the knee.

2 At the top of the leg, fan your hand outward over the buttock, applying firm pressure. Then slide your hand back down to the ankle and repeat the entire LIGHT LONG STROKING and FANNING movement at least 3 times, finishing at the top of the leg.

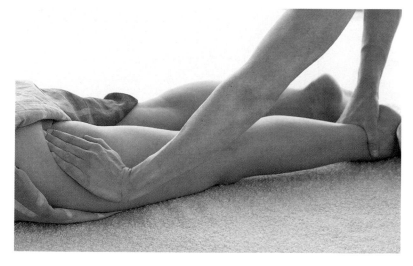

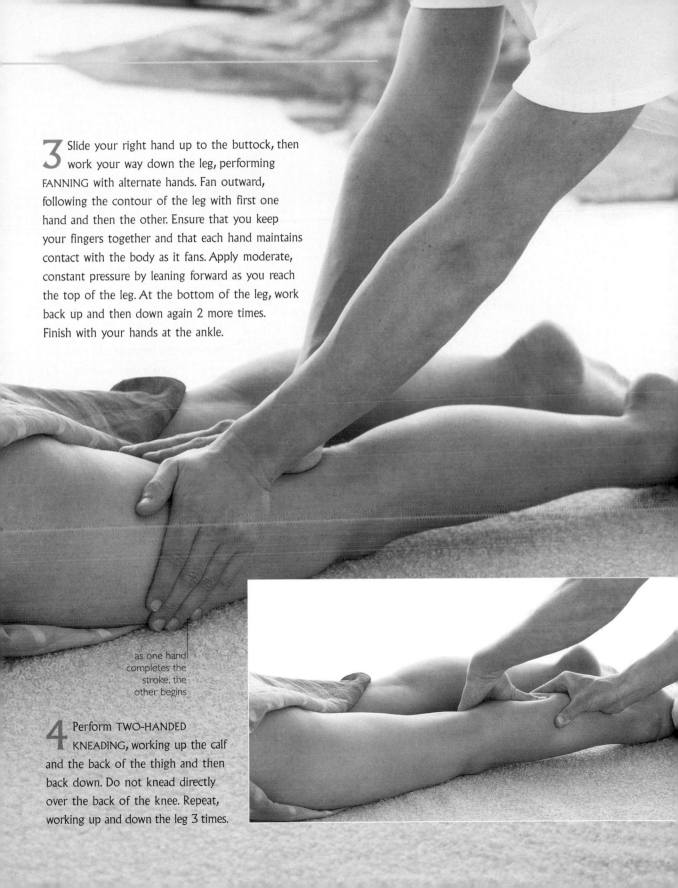

3 Slide your right hand up to the buttock, then work your way down the leg, performing FANNING with alternate hands. Fan outward, following the contour of the leg with first one hand and then the other. Ensure that you keep your fingers together and that each hand maintains contact with the body as it fans. Apply moderate, constant pressure by leaning forward as you reach the top of the leg. At the bottom of the leg, work back up and then down again 2 more times. Finish with your hands at the ankle.

as one hand completes the stroke, the other begins

4 Perform TWO-HANDED KNEADING, working up the calf and the back of the thigh and then back down. Do not knead directly over the back of the knee. Repeat, working up and down the leg 3 times.

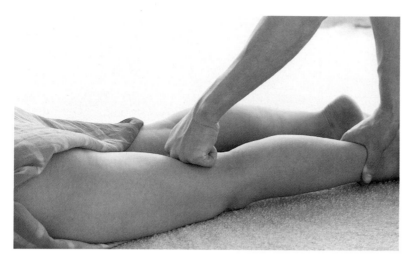

5 Hold the leg at the ankle with your right hand. Make a loose fist with your left hand and place it knuckles down on the leg, just above the back of the knee. Applying moderate pressure, perform KNUCKLE STROKING up the back of the thigh to the buttock. Repeat several times, finishing at the buttock.

6 Place your left hand flat against the buttock with fingers together, ready to perform fanning.

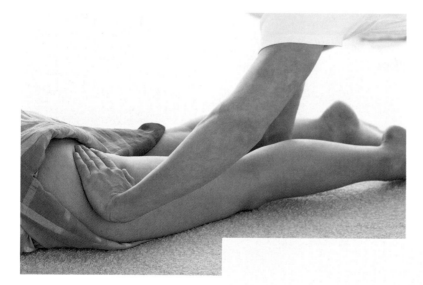

7 Perform FANNING to the buttock and the back of the thigh, working down as far as the back of the knee. Repeat, finishing with your thumb in position to stimulate the acupressure point located in the slight indent on the outer side of the buttock.

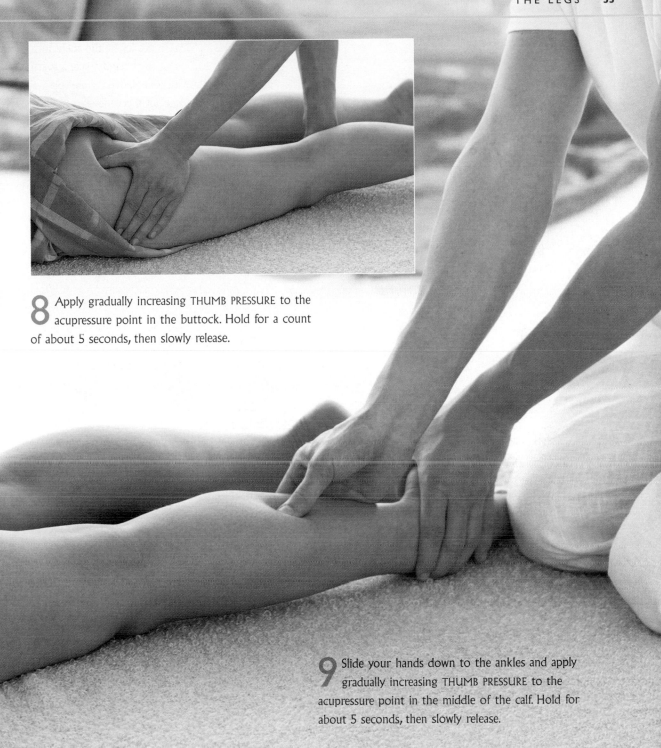

8 Apply gradually increasing THUMB PRESSURE to the
acupressure point in the buttock. Hold for a count
of about 5 seconds, then slowly release.

9 Slide your hands down to the ankles and apply
gradually increasing THUMB PRESSURE to the
acupressure point in the middle of the calf. Hold for
about 5 seconds, then slowly release.

10 Kneel a bit closer to the person. Bend the leg and rest it against your knees. Perform HAND-OVER-HAND STROKING: form your hand to the contours of the muscle and slide one hand from the bottom of the calf to the ankle, then reach down and do the same with the other hand. As one hand finishes a stroke, begin sliding the other hand up so you work in a rhythmic hand-over-hand movement. Repeat the entire movement at least 10 times.

apply moderate pressure as you stroke up the calf

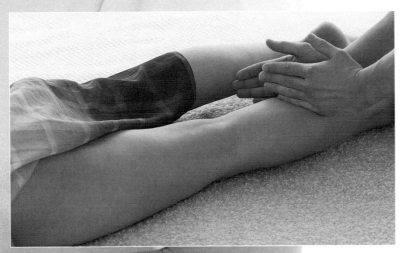

11 Replace the leg on the floor and, starting at the ankle, move up the leg, performing SAWING. Take care to keep your hands slightly curved and to maintain a brisk pace. Move up and down the leg at least 3 times, finishing at the buttock.

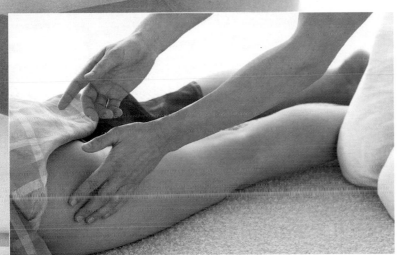

12 Work down the leg, performing FINGER TAPPING. Gently flick the skin with your fingers, keeping your hands loose and your wrists relaxed. This stimulates the nerve endings under the skin and has a pleasant, invigorating effect.

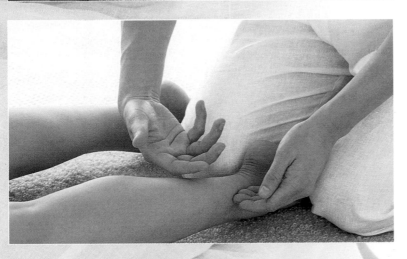

13 FINGER TAP up and down the leg at least 3 times. Then repeat the entire sequence, steps 1–13, on the other leg. Afterward, either turn the person over to continue the massage on the fronts of the legs (steps 14–20) or, if giving a full body massage, FINGER TAP over the entire back of the body before turning the person over for steps 14–20.

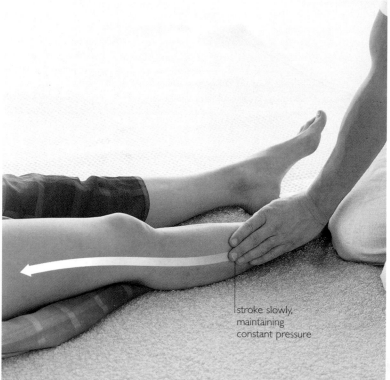

stroke slowly,
maintaining
constant pressure

14 Begin by performing LIGHT LONG STROKING along the outside of the leg, from the ankle to the top of the leg. Keep your fingers together and maintain a constant pressure as you stroke. Repeat several times.

15 Perform HEEL-OF-HAND COMPRESSIONS with one hand, working from the ankle to the knee. Use the other hand to hold the leg in position. Apply firm pressure, compressing the muscle that runs along the shin for 1–2 seconds at a time before releasing. Repeat, working up the lower leg at least 3 times.

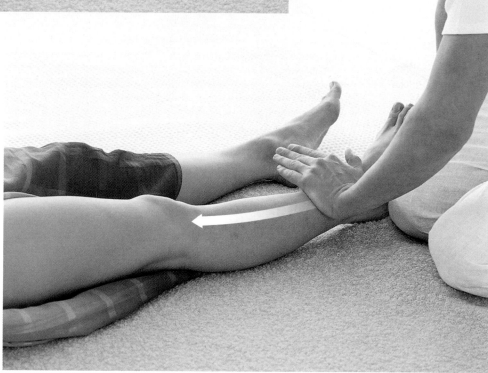

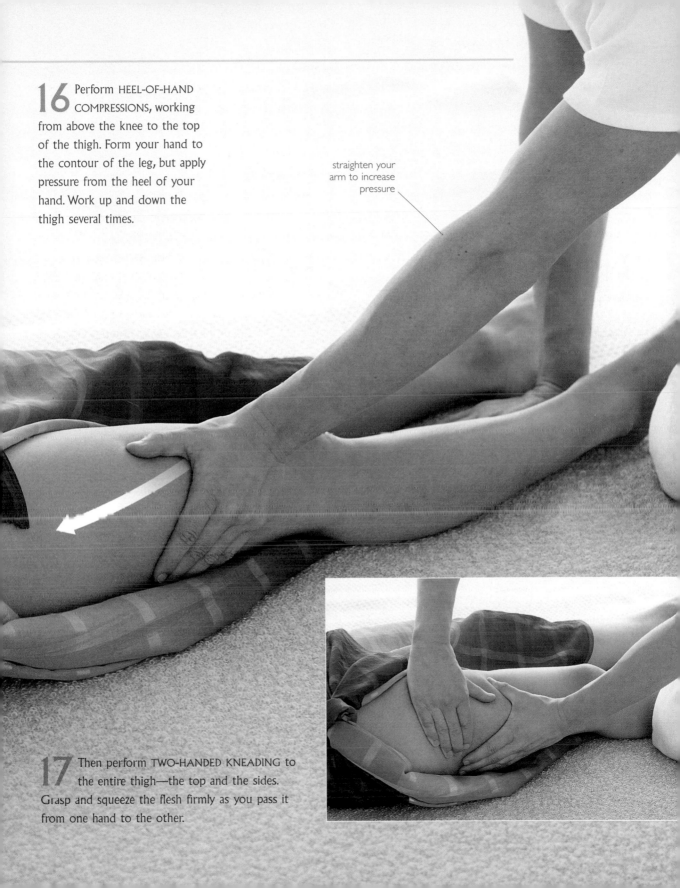

16 Perform HEEL-OF-HAND COMPRESSIONS, working from above the knee to the top of the thigh. Form your hand to the contour of the leg, but apply pressure from the heel of your hand. Work up and down the thigh several times.

straighten your arm to increase pressure

17 Then perform TWO-HANDED KNEADING to the entire thigh—the top and the sides. Grasp and squeeze the flesh firmly as you pass it from one hand to the other.

18 Move to the knee and perform THUMB PRESSURE in small circular movements, working around the kneecap. Use moderate pressure, and be sure not to probe under the kneecap—work around it.

do not apply pressure directly to the kneecap

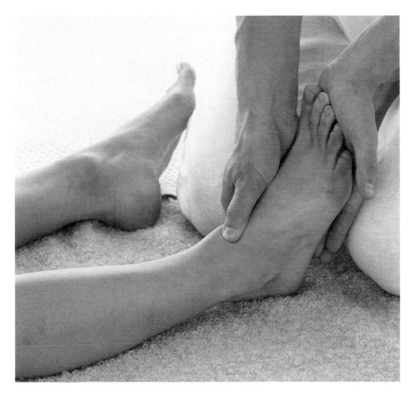

19 Gently push the foot forward with one hand. Apply gradually increasing THUMB PRESSURE to the acupressure point located in the indent at the front of the ankle. Hold for a count of 5, then gradually release.

20 Perform THUMB STRIPPING up the muscle that runs along the outside of the shin as far as the knee. Apply firm, constant pressure. Repeat, working down the leg until you've covered the whole muscle. Then repeat the entire sequence, steps 14–20, on the other leg. Finish here, or move to the feet to continue the massage.

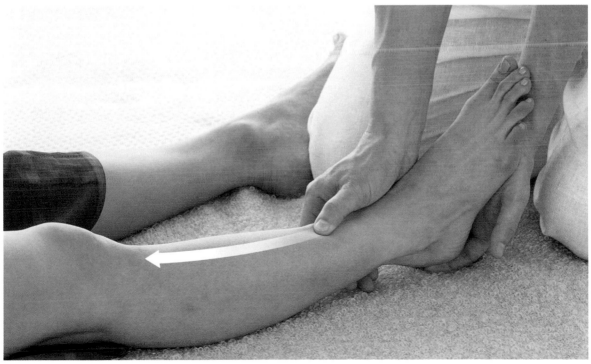

THE FEET

Remember to use a firm hand when massaging the feet—too light a touch can tickle and the experience for the recipient will be more torturous than pleasurable. If you are only massaging the feet, ensure that the person is sitting comfortably and that his or her body is well supported and completely relaxed before you begin. Take care to use the smallest amount of oil or lotion—too much will leave the feet greasy and slippery.

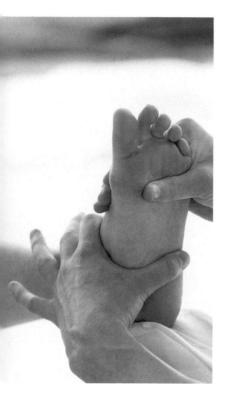 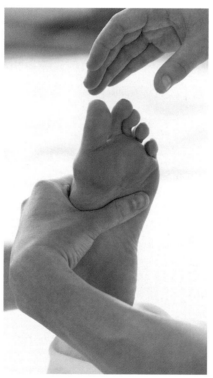 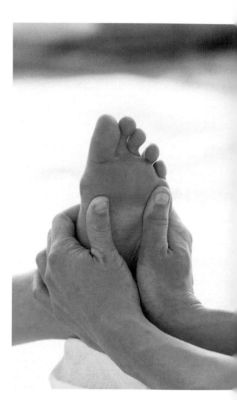

1 Grasp the foot, positioning one hand just above the heel and the other a little higher up, over the ball of the foot. Apply moderate pressure, squeezing the foot between the fingers and thumb of each hand.

2 Keep your fingers together as you firmly squeeze and pull the foot upward with one hand. Then do the same with the other hand. As one hand finishes the movement, the other moves in to take its place. Imagine stretching out an endless length of toffee. Repeat several times.

3 Grasp the foot in both hands and position your thumbs next to each other on the fleshy area at the top of the sole. Perform THUMB FANNING, stretching the foot outward. Repeat several times, moving down the foot.

4 Hold the foot by the heel with one hand. With the other hand, perform KNUCKLE FANNING to the arch of the foot. Apply firm pressure with each knuckle. This stretches and relaxes the muscles. Repeat several times.

apply pressure with your knuckles, leading with your little finger

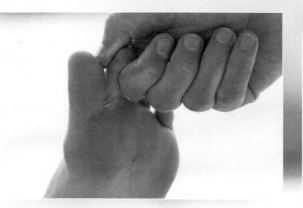

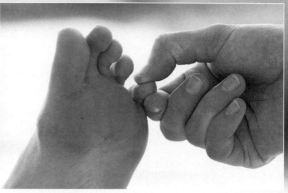

5 Starting with the big toe, take hold of each toe between your thumb and index finger and gently squeeze and pull. Be sure not to yank the toes. Pull each toe once in succession, then repeat starting at the big toe again.

6 Starting with the big toe, grasp the tip of each toe between your thumb and index finger and perform TWEAKING. Tweak each toe once in succession, then repeat starting at the big toe again.

bend foot just enough to stretch instep muscles

7 Support the foot on your knee. Gently press the toes down with one hand as you perform CROSS-FIBER FRICTION with the other. Curl your fingers slightly and gently brush your fingertips back and forth over the top of the foot. Work up toward the ankle and back again.

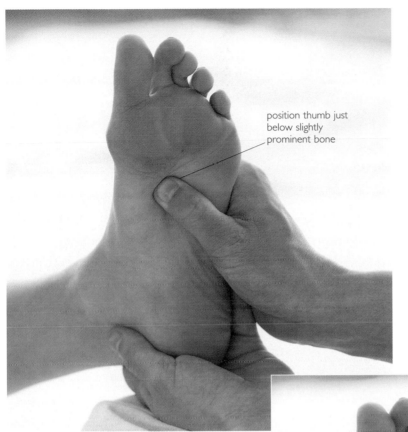

position thumb just
below slightly
prominent bone

8 Support the foot in one hand as you apply gradually increasing THUMB PRESSURE to the acupressure point just below the ball of the foot. Hold for a count of 5, then release for a count of 5. This has a deeply relaxing effect.

9 Still supporting the foot, work around the edges of it, applying CORKSCREW THUMB PRESSURE. Then repeat the entire sequence, steps 1–9, on the other foot. To finish, gently squeeze both feet simultaneously in each of your hands. If you are just giving a foot massage, finish here; otherwise move up and kneel by the person's right side, ready to begin work on the arms and hands.

THE ARMS AND HANDS

People will often try to help you by holding up their arms for you to massage, but this only causes them to tense their muscles. To encourage the person to relax his or her arm, hold the hand in your hand and gently swing the arm back and forth until it feels heavier. When massaging, do not work the inside of the elbow intensively; glide over the arteries and veins that are close to the surface of the skin here. Generally, the rule is to massage up the arm, toward the lymph glands in the armpit.

1 Kneel on the person's right side and take hold of the right hand in your right hand as if to shake it. With your other hand, lightly stroke in one smooth movement up the entire length of the arm to the shoulder.

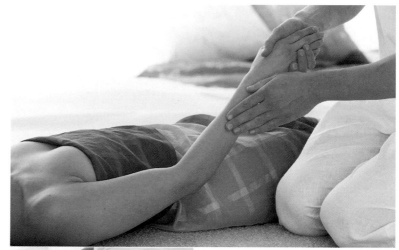

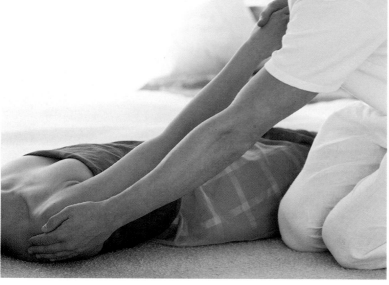

2 Stroke over the shoulder, cupping your hand over it, then lightly stroke back down the arm to the wrist, ready to perform the entire stroke again. The thrust of the movement is in the downward stroke. Repeat several times.

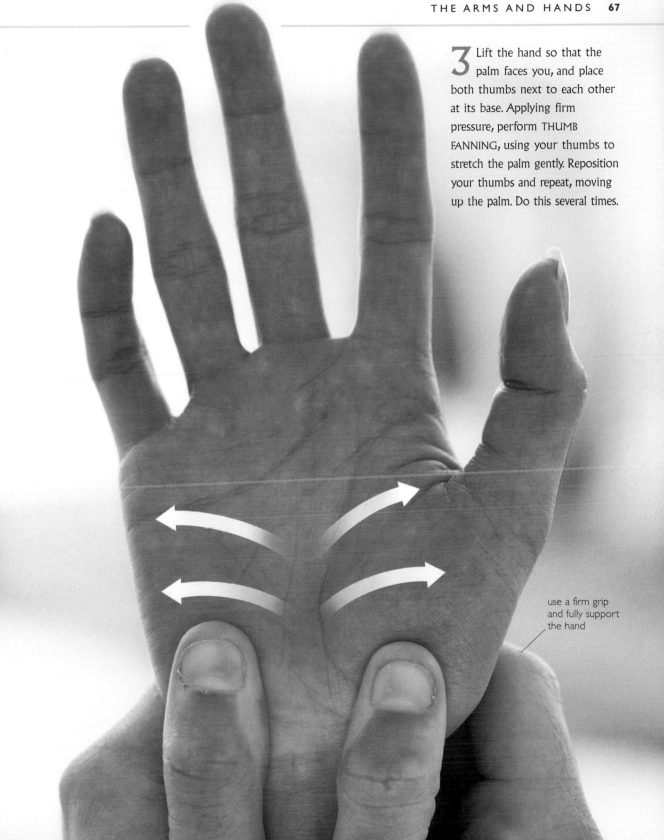

3 Lift the hand so that the palm faces you, and place both thumbs next to each other at its base. Applying firm pressure, perform THUMB FANNING, using your thumbs to stretch the palm gently. Reposition your thumbs and repeat, moving up the palm. Do this several times.

use a firm grip and fully support the hand

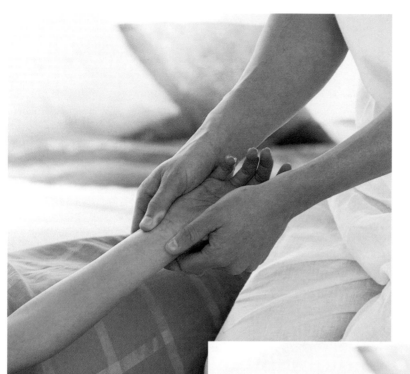

4 Lower the hand, then turn the arm outward so that the palm faces upward. Support the hand in your hands, and place your thumbs next to each other on the wrist. Perform THUMB FANNING, sliding your thumbs outward across the tendons and muscle fibers. Work up as far as the delicate area on the inside of the elbow, then slide your thumbs back down to the wrist and repeat at least 2 more times.

5 Take hold of the person's hand as if to shake it, and turn the arm inward. With your left hand, perform ONE-HANDED KNEADING up the forearm, gently squeezing the flesh between your thumb and fingers. At the top of the forearm, slide your hand back down the arm to the wrist and repeat. At the end of the final kneading stroke, your left thumb is in position on the fleshy area at the top of the elbow, ready to apply thumb pressure.

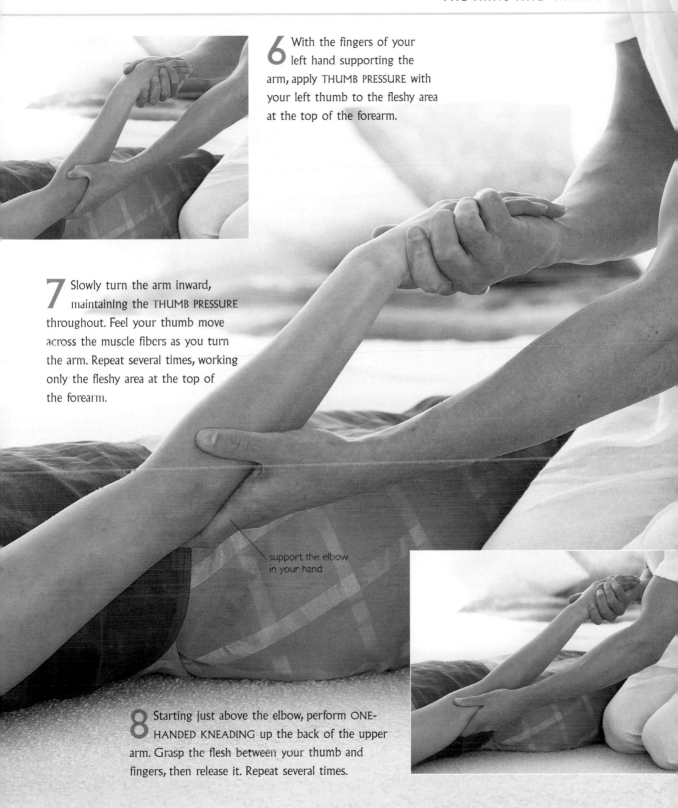

6 With the fingers of your left hand supporting the arm, apply THUMB PRESSURE with your left thumb to the fleshy area at the top of the forearm.

7 Slowly turn the arm inward, maintaining the THUMB PRESSURE throughout. Feel your thumb move across the muscle fibers as you turn the arm. Repeat several times, working only the fleshy area at the top of the forearm.

support the elbow in your hand

8 Starting just above the elbow, perform ONE-HANDED KNEADING up the back of the upper arm. Grasp the flesh between your thumb and fingers, then release it. Repeat several times.

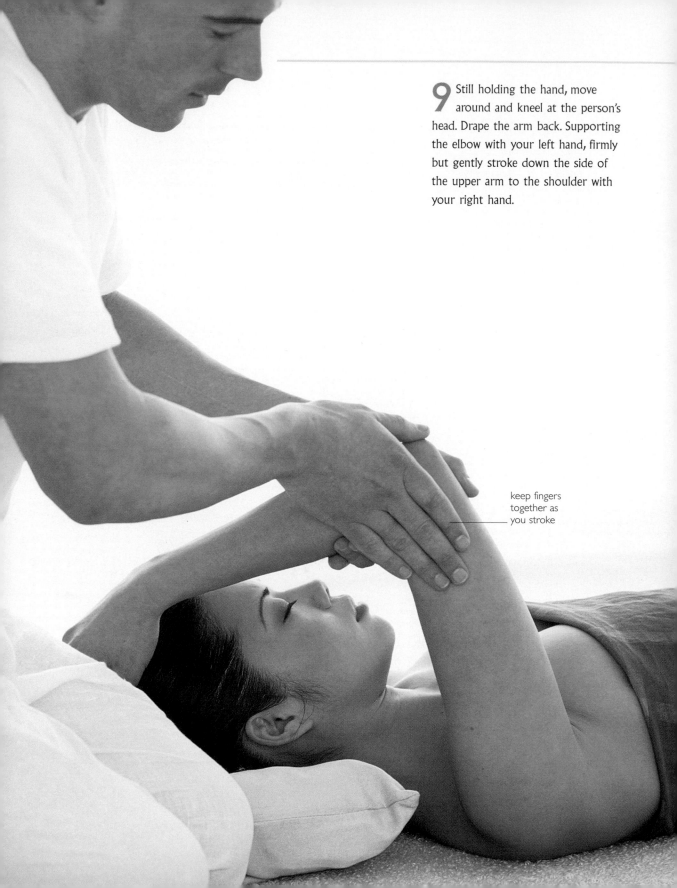

9 Still holding the hand, move around and kneel at the person's head. Drape the arm back. Supporting the elbow with your left hand, firmly but gently stroke down the side of the upper arm to the shoulder with your right hand.

keep fingers together as you stroke

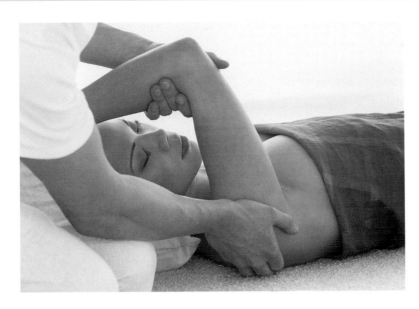

10 Cup the shoulder with your right hand, then trail your fingers back up the biceps to the elbow. Stroke the entire arm several times.

11 Lift the arm to straighten it slightly. Perform LIFTING by firmly pressing the biceps with your right palm, then grasping it between your fingers and thumb and gently pulling and squeezing it. Release and repeat several times. Replace the arm by the side of the body, and perform steps 1–11 on the left arm.

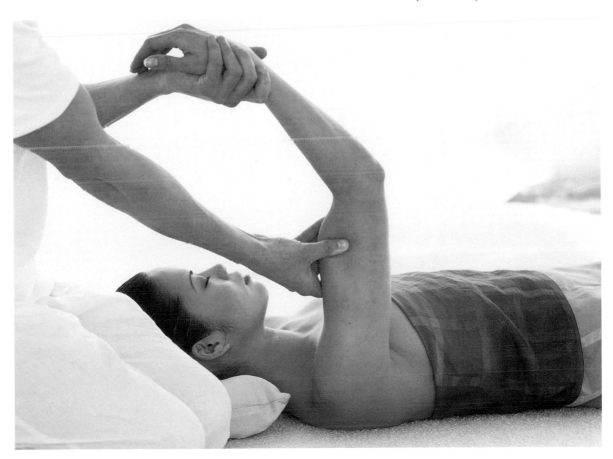

THE TORSO

People often feel awkward about massaging the torso, especially when working on women. This routine works for both men and women. Remember to keep the pressure moderate to light when massaging the abdomen; the rib cage encases the heart and lungs, but only muscle protects the vital organs in the abdominal area. I recommend that you avoid massaging the abdomen for at least one hour after a heavy meal. It is safe to perform this massage very gently on a pregnant woman in her second or third trimester.

1 Kneel at the person's side and lean over to work on the side furthest from you. Start by placing both hands next to each other on the side of the body. Stroke up toward you with one hand, applying gentle to moderate pressure to the side and abdomen. As your hand comes off the body, begin stroking up with the other hand. Stroke toward you in a continuous rhythm, with each hand reaching over to take the place of the other as it completes a stroke. Then move around to the other side of the person and repeat.

apply pressure as you stroke

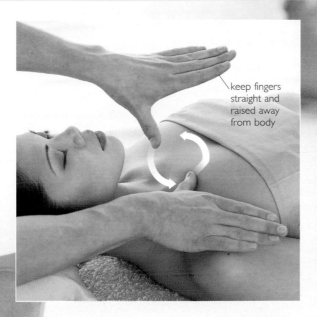

keep fingers
straight and
raised away
from body

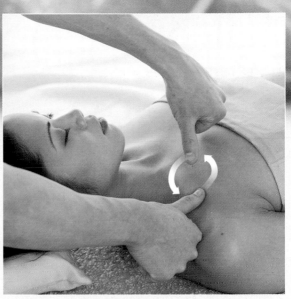

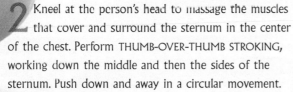

2 Kneel at the person's head to massage the muscles that cover and surround the sternum in the center of the chest. Perform THUMB-OVER-THUMB STROKING, working down the middle and then the sides of the sternum. Push down and away in a circular movement.

3 Then perform THUMB-OVER-THUMB STROKING, working along the muscles on the underside of the collar bone. Push toward the shoulder with each thumb movement. Work along the collar bone at least 3 times, then repeat on the other side.

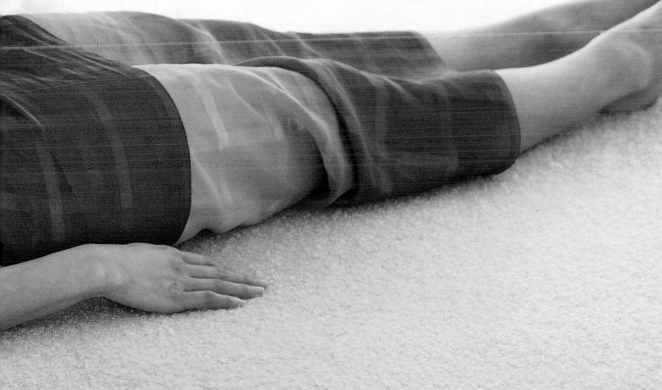

THE NECK AND SHOULDERS

Muscle strain and stiffness in the neck and shoulders can occur as a result of stress that causes you to tense the area, or from simply holding an awkward position, for example when working at a computer. During this massage, you cradle and support the head, taking the pressure off the muscles in the neck and shoulders. Ask the person to use your hands as a pillow. I find that this is a much more effective technique for inducing relaxation than simply asking a person to relax.

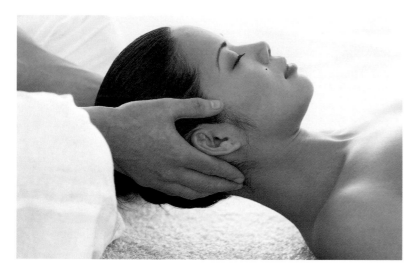

1 Sit cross-legged behind the person and cradle his or her head in your hands. Position your fingers just under the bony ridge at the base of the skull and gently pull the head toward you, stretching the muscles in the neck. Hold for about 10 seconds, then gently release. Take care not to bend the neck or tilt the head too far forward.

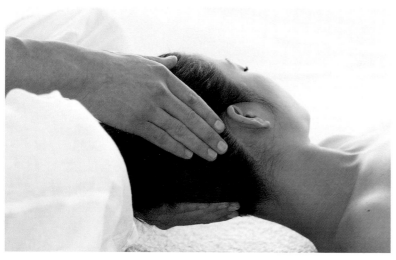

2 Keeping the neck straight, gently turn the head to the left and cradle it in your left hand. Position your left hand just behind the person's ear, not over it, with your thumb and index finger on either side of it. Use your leg as a support to steady your arm.

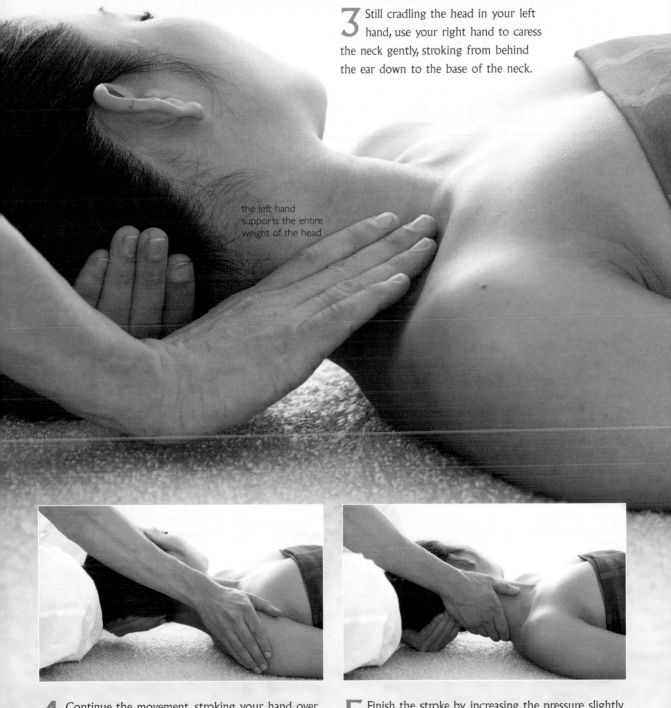

3 Still cradling the head in your left hand, use your right hand to caress the neck gently, stroking from behind the ear down to the base of the neck.

the left hand supports the entire weight of the head

4 Continue the movement, stroking your hand over and then underneath the shoulder. Form your hand to the contour of the shoulder.

5 Finish the stroke by increasing the pressure slightly as you glide up the neck to the base of the skull. Repeat the entire stroke, steps 3–5, at least 3 times.

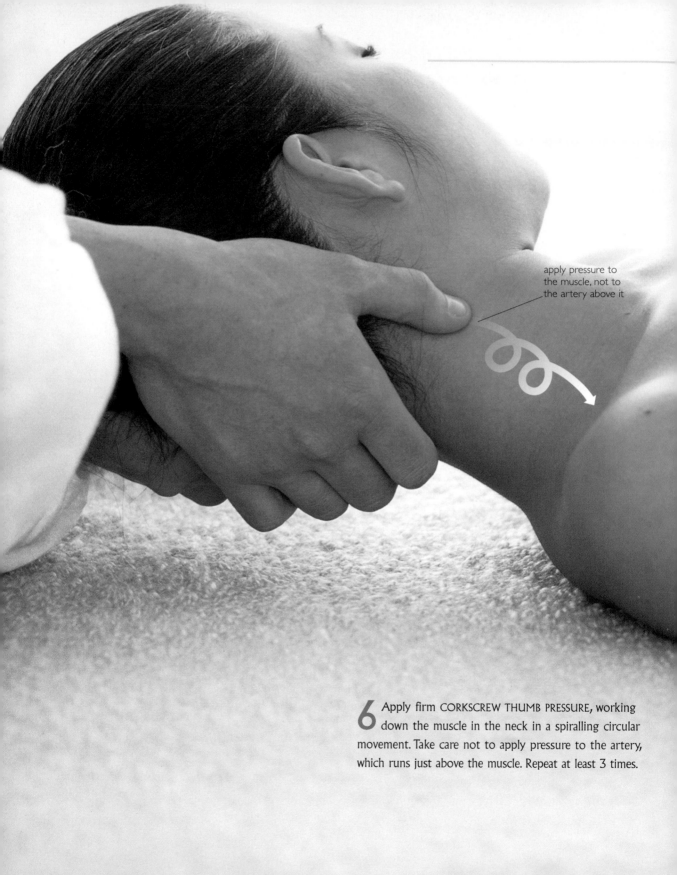

apply pressure to
the muscle, not to
the artery above it

6 Apply firm CORKSCREW THUMB PRESSURE, working
down the muscle in the neck in a spiralling circular
movement. Take care not to apply pressure to the artery,
which runs just above the muscle. Repeat at least 3 times.

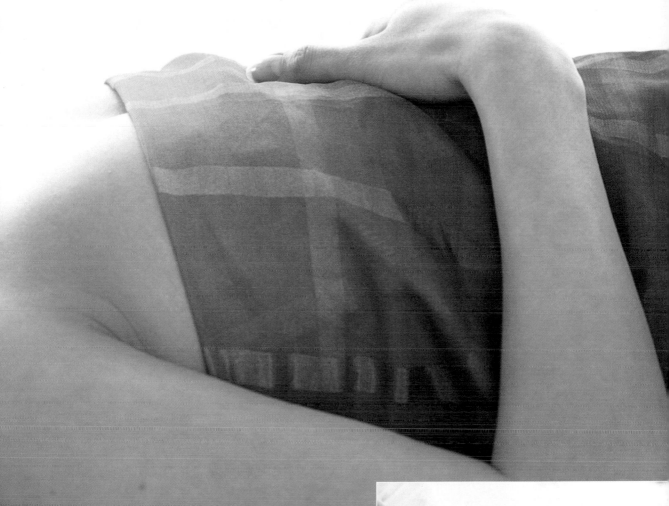

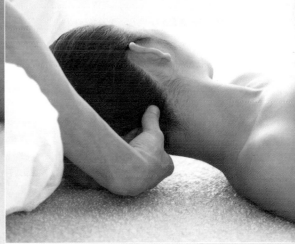

7 Apply firm CORKSCREW THUMB PRESSURE along the bony ridge at the base of the skull. Work slowly, feeling for tense muscles. Then turn the head back to the right, cradling it in your right hand. Repeat steps 3–7 on the left side of the neck, then return the head to the center. To end the session, you might want to place a folded towel or a small cushion under the neck as a support and allow the person to relax for a minute or two.

QUICK REFERENCE

Once you become familiar with the sequence of strokes that makes up the full body massage, use these quick-reference charts to help you to flow seamlessly from one movement to the next. Remember, you can use the whole routine or just part of it. Focus more attention on tense areas.

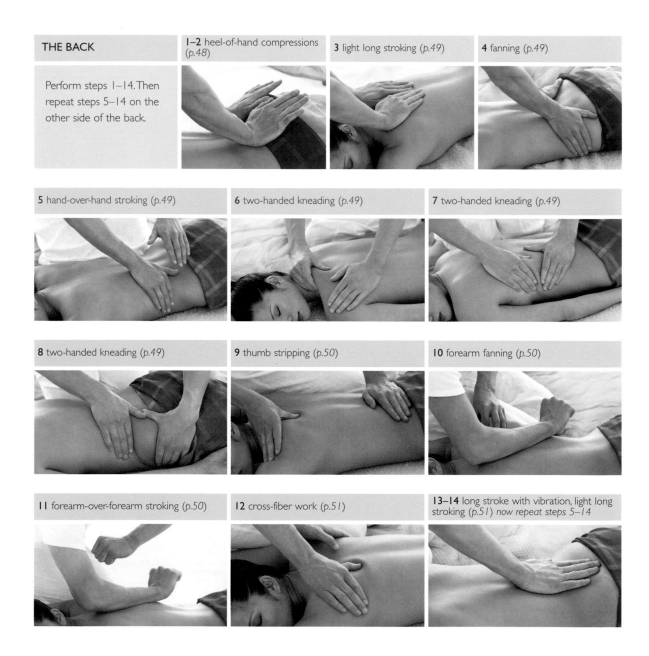

THE BACK

Perform steps 1–14. Then repeat steps 5–14 on the other side of the back.

1–2 heel-of-hand compressions (*p.48*)

3 light long stroking (*p.49*)

4 fanning (*p.49*)

5 hand-over-hand stroking (*p.49*)

6 two-handed kneading (*p.49*)

7 two-handed kneading (*p.49*)

8 two-handed kneading (*p.49*)

9 thumb stripping (*p.50*)

10 forearm fanning (*p.50*)

11 forearm-over-forearm stroking (*p.50*)

12 cross-fiber work (*p.51*)

13–14 long stroke with vibration, light long stroking (*p.51*) *now repeat steps 5–14*

THE LEGS

Complete steps 1–13, then repeat on the other leg. Turn the person over and perform steps 14–20 on one leg, then on the other.

1–2 light long stroking with fanning (p.52)

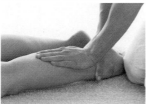

3 fanning with alternate hands (p.53)

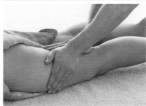

4 two-handed kneading (p.53)

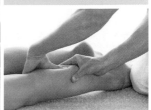

5 knuckle stroking (p.54)

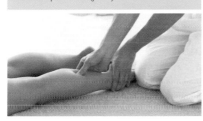

6–7 fanning (p.54)

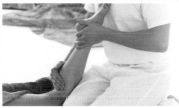

8 thumb pressure (p.55)

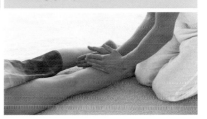

9 thumb pressure (p.55)

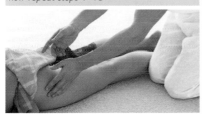

10 hand-over-hand stroking (p.56)

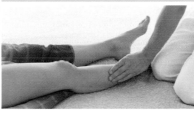

11 sawing (p.57)

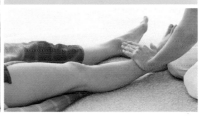

12–13 finger tapping (p.57)
now repeat steps 1–13

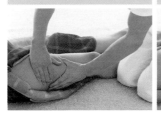

14 light long stroking (p.58)

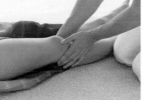

15–16 heel-of-hand compressions (p.58)

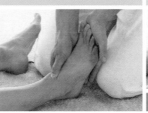

17 two-handed kneading (p.59)

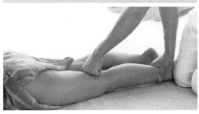

18 circular thumb pressure (p.60)

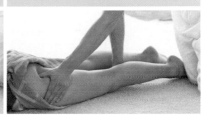

19 thumb pressure (p.61)

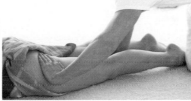

20 thumb stripping (p.61)
now repeat steps14–20

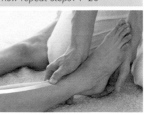

THE FEET

Complete this sequence, then repeat it on the other foot.

1–2 pulling and squeezing (*p.62*)

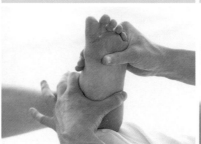

3 thumb fanning (*p.62*)

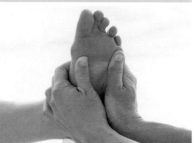

4 knuckle fanning (*p.63*)

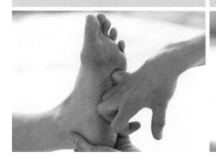

5 pulling (*p.64*)

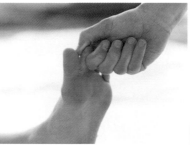

6 tweaking (*p.64*)

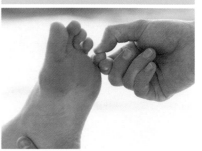

7 cross-fiber friction (*p.64*)

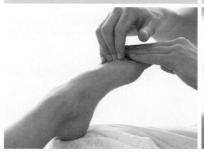

8 thumb pressure (*p.65*)

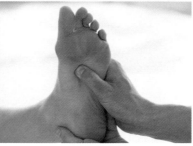

9 corkscrew thumb pressure (*p.65*)
now repeat steps 1–9

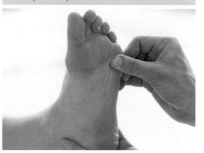

THE ARMS AND HANDS

Complete this sequence, then repeat it on the other arm and hand.

1–2 stroking (*p.66*)

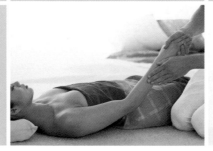

3 thumb fanning (*p.67*)

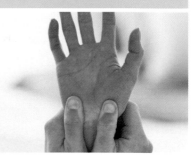

4 thumb fanning (*p.68*)

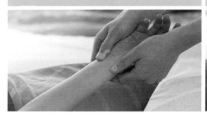

5 one-handed kneading (*p.68*)

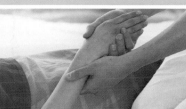

6–7 thumb pressure with arm turn (*p.69*)

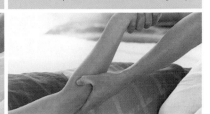

8 one-handed kneading (*p.69*)

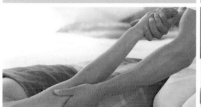

9–10 stroking (*pp.70–71*)

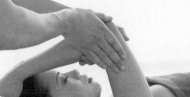

11 lifting (*p.71*)
now repeat steps 1–11

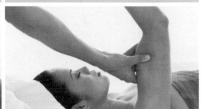

THE TORSO

Perform step 1, then move around and repeat the stroke on the other side of the body before completing the sequence.

1 hand-over-hand stroking (*p.72*)
now repeat on the other side

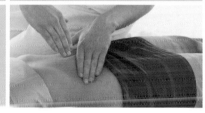

2 thumb-over-thumb stroking (*p.73*)

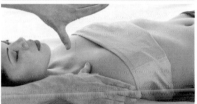

3 thumb-over-thumb stroking (*p.73*)

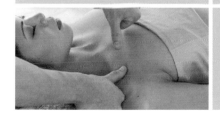

THE NECK AND SHOULDERS

At the end of this sequence, go back and repeat steps 3–7 on the other side of the neck.

1–2 cradling and tugging (*p.74*)

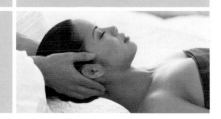

3–5 stroking (*p.75*)

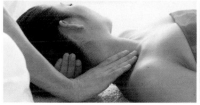

6 corkscrew thumb pressure (*p.76*)

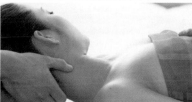

7 corkscrew thumb pressure (*p.77*)
now repeat steps 3–7

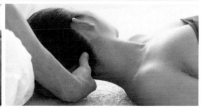

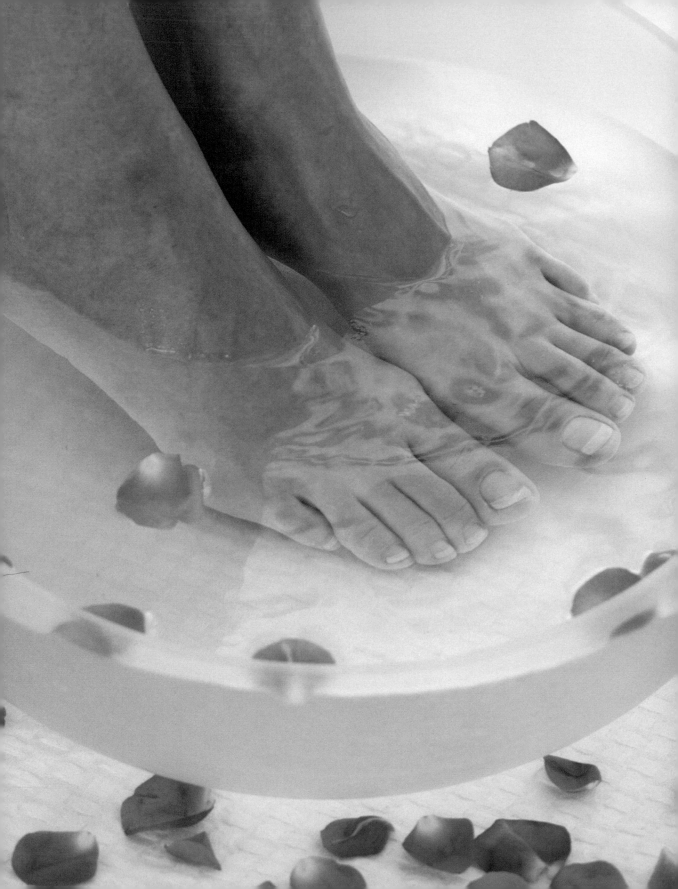

PAMPERING SPA ROUTINES

Here I present a selection of my favorite luxurious, head-to-toe spa routines. Try a Cleansing Facial to leave skin refreshed and radiant, or a Papaya Wrap to smooth and moisturize the whole body. Experiment with the numerous beauty recipes for everything from a fresh grape conditioner for lustrous, shiny locks to an indulgent kiwi foot mask. Treat a friend to any of the sumptuous routines that follow and, with any luck, they'll treat you too.

CLEANSING FACIAL

Many of my older clients attribute their youthful good looks to regular facial massages. This profoundly relaxing treatment cleanses the skin, tones the facial muscles, and boosts the circulation to give a glowing and radiant complexion. Use your regular cleanser or a drop or two of a light oil, such as sweet almond. If using oil, use an astringent such as the one suggested below to cleanse the face after the treatment. Sit cross-legged with the person lying on their back, their head cradled in your lap.

TIPS FOR FACIALS
• Perform weekly cleansing facials to reduce the appearance of blackheads and prevent pores from becoming blocked.
• Keep nails short to avoid scratching the delicate facial skin.
• If the person wears contact lenses, these must be removed before beginning this treatment.

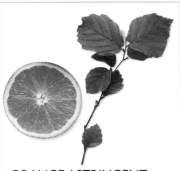

ORANGE ASTRINGENT
• 1 tsp Epsom salts
• 1 tbsp witch hazel
• 8 tbsp distilled water
• 1 drop orange, rose, or lavender essential oil

Mix the ingredients together in a small bottle, and shake gently until the Epsom salts have completely dissolved.

Try using this astringent as a facial spritzer in the summer. A quick spray instantly cools, cleanses, and refreshes. Small spritzer bottles are readily available from beauty suppliers and larger drug stores.

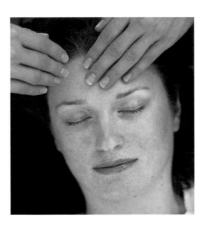

1 Gently stroke across the forehead, using alternate hands. Repeat several times.

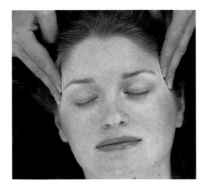

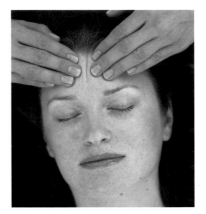

2 Starting between the eyebrows, apply FINGER PRESSURE in small circular movements, working from the eyebrows to the hairline. Reposition your hands; repeat, moving outward.

3 Place two fingers on each temple and apply light FINGER PRESSURE in small circular movements. Do this for at least 30 seconds.

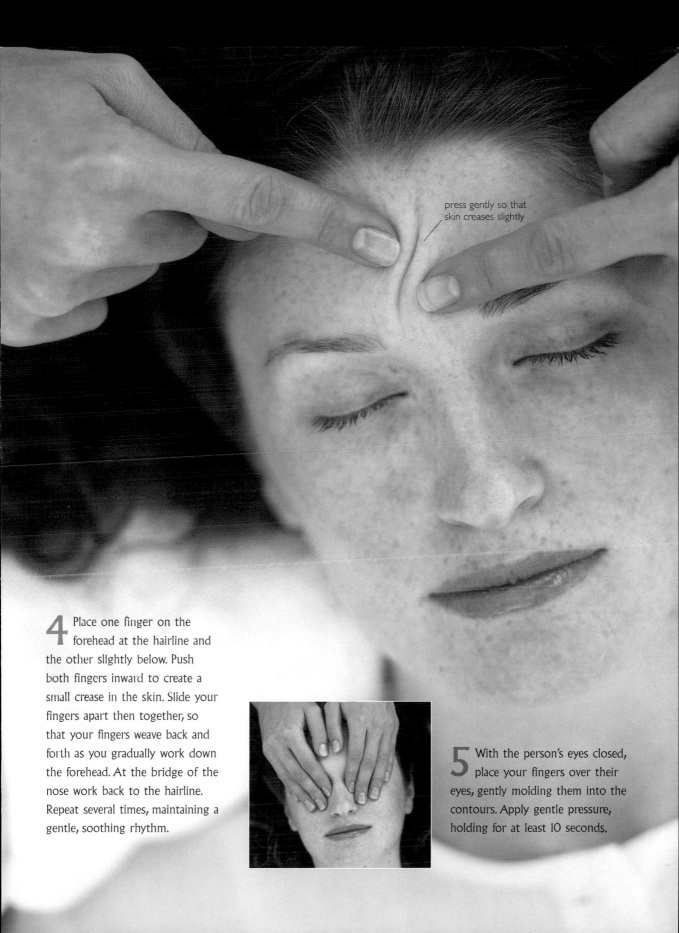

press gently so that
skin creases slightly

4 Place one finger on the
forehead at the hairline and
the other slightly below. Push
both fingers inward to create a
small crease in the skin. Slide your
fingers apart then together, so
that your fingers weave back and
forth as you gradually work down
the forehead. At the bridge of the
nose work back to the hairline.
Repeat several times, maintaining a
gentle, soothing rhythm.

5 With the person's eyes closed,
place your fingers over their
eyes, gently molding them into the
contours. Apply gentle pressure,
holding for at least 10 seconds.

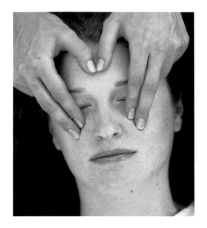
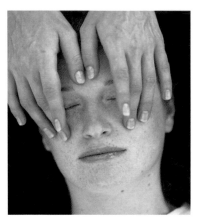
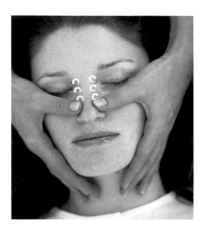

6 Use one or two fingers to apply FINGER PRESSURE, working in small circular movements, to the bony ridge along the bottom of the eye. Work back and forth at least 3 times.

7 Perform gentle TAPPING under the eyes, quickly alternating between your index and middle fingers to create a vibrating effect. Tap with the soft pads of your fingers.

8 Apply THUMB PRESSURE along the sides of the nose, working in small circular movements. Work up the nose at least 3 times.

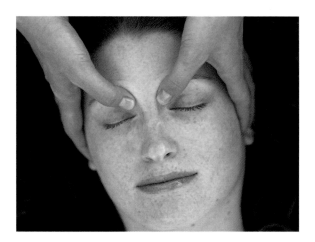
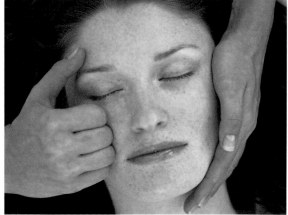

9 Apply gradually increasing THUMB PRESSURE to the acupressure point at the top of the nose. Press inward toward the bridge of the nose. Hold for a count of 5, then release for a count of 5.

10 Make a loose fist and place your knuckles on the cheek with your thumb pointing toward you in position for KNUCKLE FANNING. Cradle the face with your other hand.

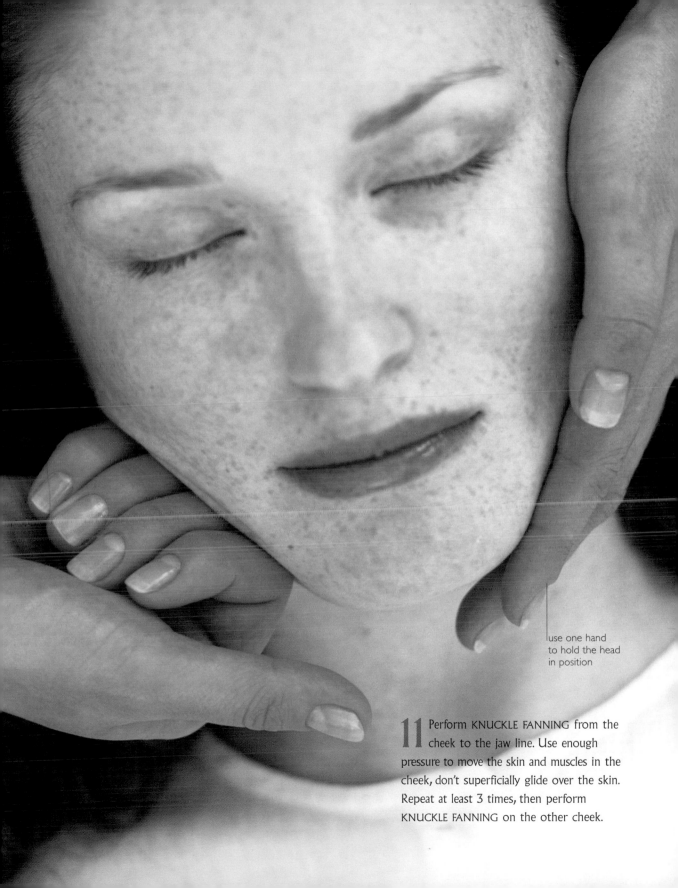

use one hand
to hold the head
in position

11 Perform KNUCKLE FANNING from the
cheek to the jaw line. Use enough
pressure to move the skin and muscles in the
cheek, don't superficially glide over the skin.
Repeat at least 3 times, then perform
KNUCKLE FANNING on the other cheek.

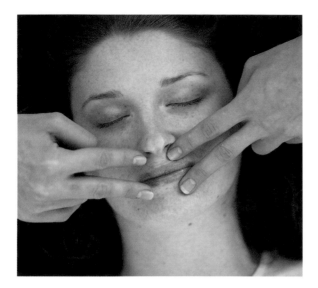

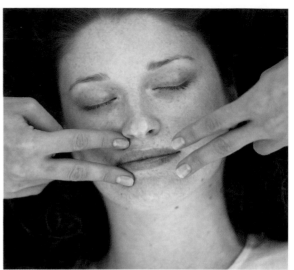

12 Making a V-shape with your fingers, position one finger above the mouth and one below. With one hand, gently stroke across the mouth from one cheek to the other.

13 As you finish the stroke and begin to lift your fingers away, stroke across from one side of the mouth to the other with your other hand. Repeat several times, maintaining a soothing, rhythmic pace.

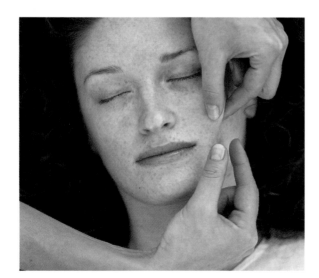

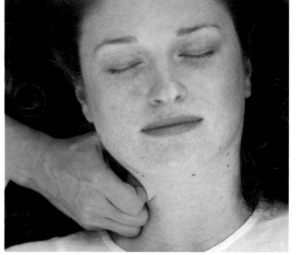

14 Grasp a small fold of skin on the cheek between thumb and forefinger, gently tweak it, then release. Perform TWEAKING with alternate hands, moving around the cheek. Keep the movements gentle but brisk, taking care not to pinch. Perform about 60 tweaks per cheek.

15 Place your thumb behind the neck and use this to help control the pressure as you perform KNUCKLE FANNING. Gently fan your knuckles forward, working down the side of the neck. Position your other hand and repeat on the other side of the neck.

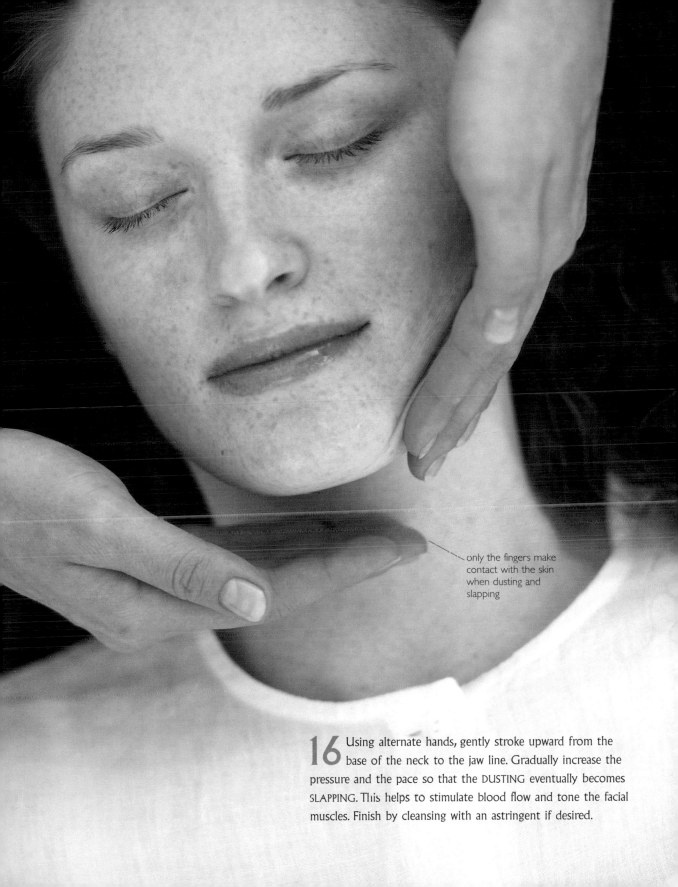

only the fingers make
contact with the skin
when dusting and
slapping

16 Using alternate hands, gently stroke upward from the base of the neck to the jaw line. Gradually increase the pressure and the pace so that the DUSTING eventually becomes SLAPPING. This helps to stimulate blood flow and tone the facial muscles. Finish by cleansing with an astringent if desired.

AMAZING SCALP MASSAGE

During a scalp treatment, the aim is to massage the thin layer of muscles that cover the skull and to stimulate blood flow to the area. This soothing massage is also an effective headache treatment. You use your fingertips to perform this massage, so be sure to check that your fingernails are short. Use gentle to moderate pressure, just enough to move the scalp. As the muscles in the face and scalp relax, the scalp will move more easily. Don't use any oil or lotion for this massage.

FRESH GRAPE CONDITIONER

Try following your normal shampooing routine with this intensive hair conditioning treatment:
Purée 4oz (125g) grapes with seeds in a food processor, or crush in a pestle and mortar. Apply the mixture, starting at the scalp and working into the hair. Cover with a shower cap, leave for 20 minutes, then rinse off.

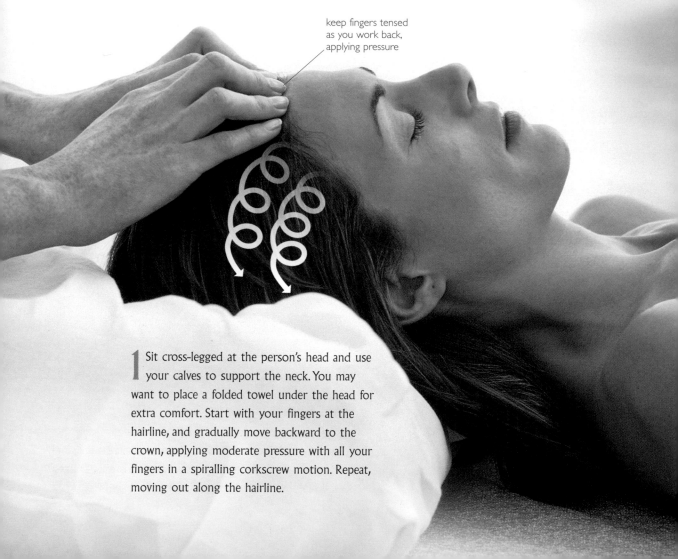

keep fingers tensed as you work back, applying pressure

1 Sit cross-legged at the person's head and use your calves to support the neck. You may want to place a folded towel under the head for extra comfort. Start with your fingers at the hairline, and gradually move backward to the crown, applying moderate pressure with all your fingers in a spiralling corkscrew motion. Repeat, moving out along the hairline.

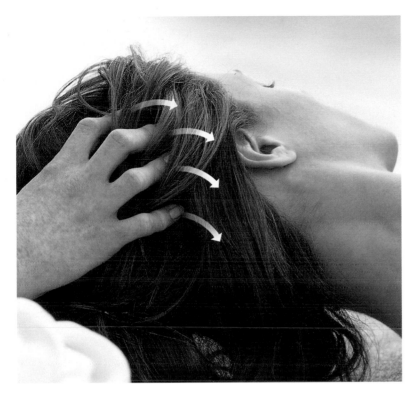

2 Gently turn the head to the left, carefully supporting it in your left hand. Position your right thumb at the back of the head as an anchor and perform FINGER FANNING on the side of the head. Repeat, moving forward to the hairline, covering the whole side of the head.

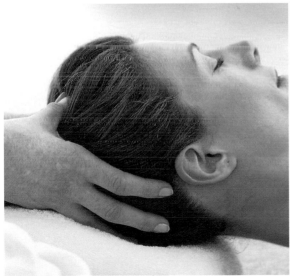

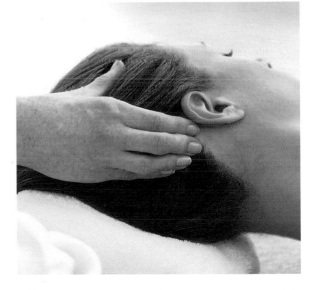

3 Turn the head back to the center and, supporting it in your hands, position your fingers behind the ears and your thumbs at the crown. Apply firm THUMB PRESSURE to the entire crown area.

4 Turn the head to the left, supporting it in your left hand. Using your right thumb as a support, use all four fingers to apply FINGER PRESSURE in small circular movements under the bony ridge at the base of the skull.

5 Turn the head back to the center and, with fingertips positioned along the bony ridge at the base of the skull, support the weight of the head. Curl your fingers slightly and feel the head become heavy as the muscles in the scalp and neck relax.

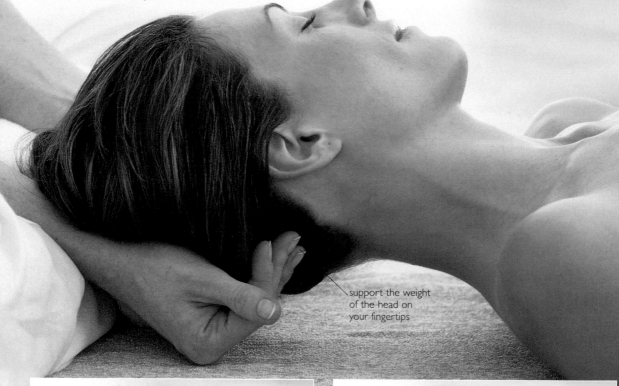

support the weight
of the head on
your fingertips

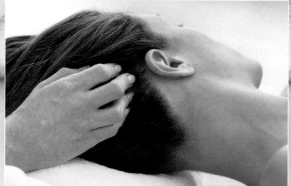

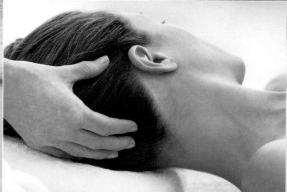

6 Gently roll the head to the left. Position your right hand behind the ear with your thumb against the head and fingers slightly curled.

7 Keeping your thumb in the same position, perform FINGER FANNING downward, following the shape of the head. Repeat several times, then gently roll the head to the right and repeat steps 2–7 on the other side.

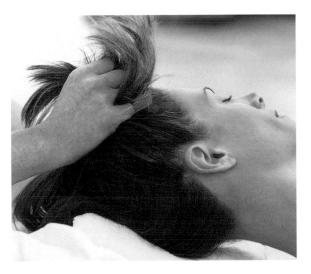

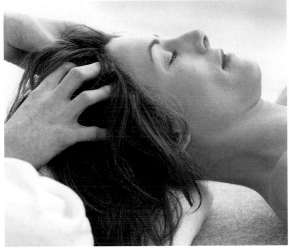

8 Turn the head back to center. Grasp a handful of hair and gently tug it hard enough to move the scalp slightly but not to cause pain. Repeat, moving around the head, tugging different handfuls of hair.

9 Finish by scratching the scalp, rubbing your fingertips all over the head, gently tousling the hair. This is an invigorating finishing move.

SELF-MASSAGE FOR THE SCALP

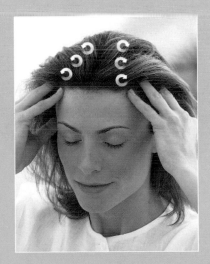

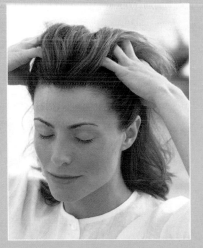

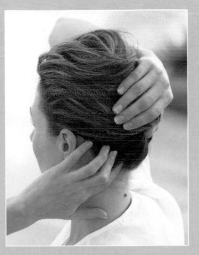

1 Place your fingers at your hairline. Apply FINGER PRESSURE, working backward in small circles toward the crown. Repeat several times.

2 Tense your fingers slightly and, starting at the hairline, rake backward through the hair. Repeat several times, raking the whole head.

3 Work along the ridge at the base of your skull, applying FINGER PRESSURE in small circles. Repeat on the other side of the head.

ROSE HAND TREATMENT

People often don't realize just how much tension accumulates in the hands, especially if they work with their hands, or if they type. This sublime hand massage can help to prevent muscle complaints such as repetitive strain injury because it increases blood flow to the hands, helping to clear adhesions that form on muscles and tendons as a result of repetitive actions. Use the rose lotion below for the massage; include fresh rose petals in the last stage of the treatment to add a hint of luxury.

TIPS FOR MOISTURIZING

• To nourish nails and moisturize cuticles, try massaging them with one drop each of rose essential oil. Cuticles can then be gently pushed back with a cotton bud.
• Apply the rose intensive moisturizing lotion below to dry skin on other parts of the body, especially the elbows, knees, and feet.

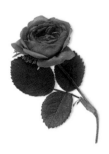

ROSE LOTION

• 1 fl oz (30ml) unscented moisturizing lotion

• 6 drops oil such as sweet almond or grapeseed

• 6–7 drops rose essential oil

Mix the ingredients together in a bowl or bottle.

Also needed:

• 2 large pieces plastic wrap to wrap around hands

• 1 towel and 2 oven mits or 2 towels

• 2 handfuls fresh rose petals (optional)

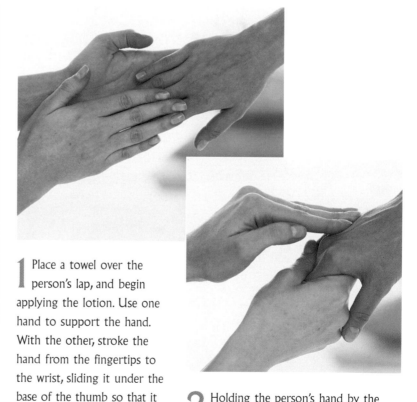

1 Place a towel over the person's lap, and begin applying the lotion. Use one hand to support the hand. With the other, stroke the hand from the fingertips to the wrist, sliding it under the base of the thumb so that it then supports the hand. Repeat with both hands in a hand-over-hand movement.

2 Holding the person's hand by the fingers, perform CROSS-FIBER FRICTION. Sweep your fingertips back and forth across the tendons on the top of the hand, maintaining a swift but rhythmic pace.

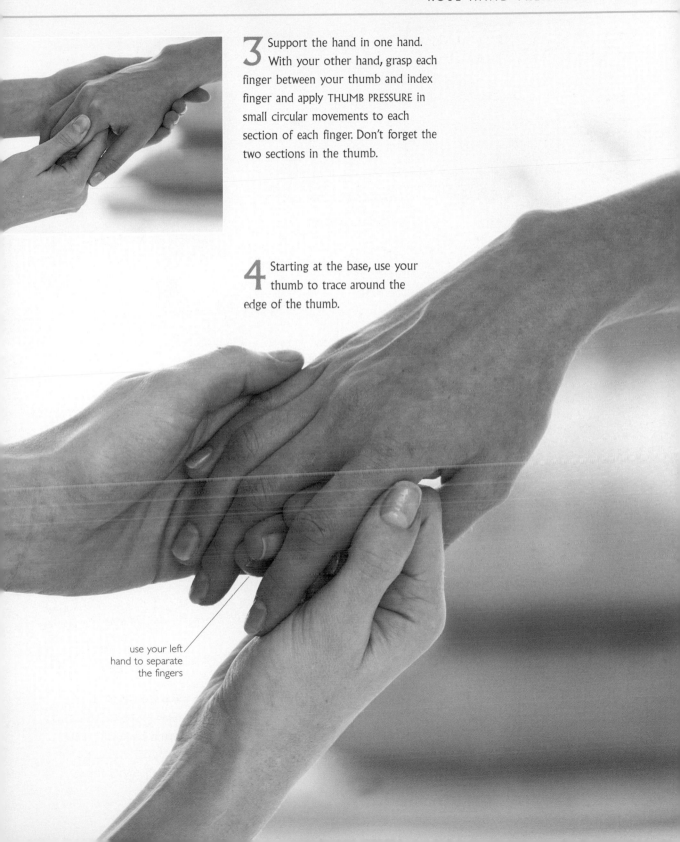

3 Support the hand in one hand. With your other hand, grasp each finger between your thumb and index finger and apply THUMB PRESSURE in small circular movements to each section of each finger. Don't forget the two sections in the thumb.

4 Starting at the base, use your thumb to trace around the edge of the thumb.

use your left hand to separate the fingers

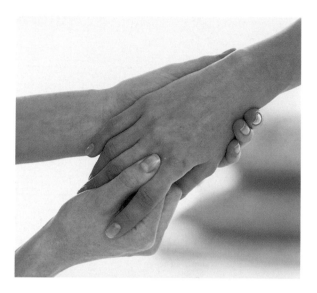

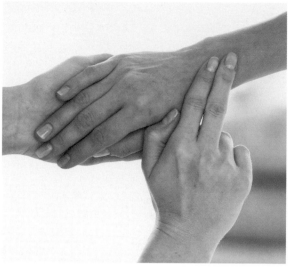

5 Then apply gentle THUMB PRESSURE to the web of skin between each of the fingers.

6 With your first two fingers, work across the bony area on top of the wrist applying FINGER PRESSURE, working in small circular movements.

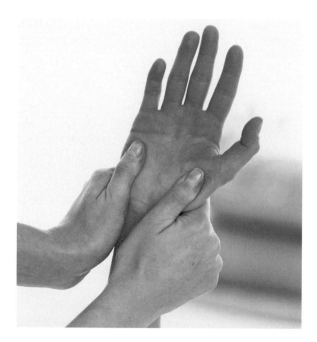

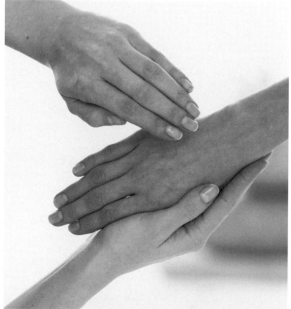

7 Turn the palm to face you and, placing your thumbs on the fleshy outer edges, gently stretch it. Reposition your thumbs and repeat, moving up the palm.

8 Finish the massage by gently but briskly TAPPING the back of the hand to stimulate the nerve endings. Then repeat steps 1–8 on the other hand.

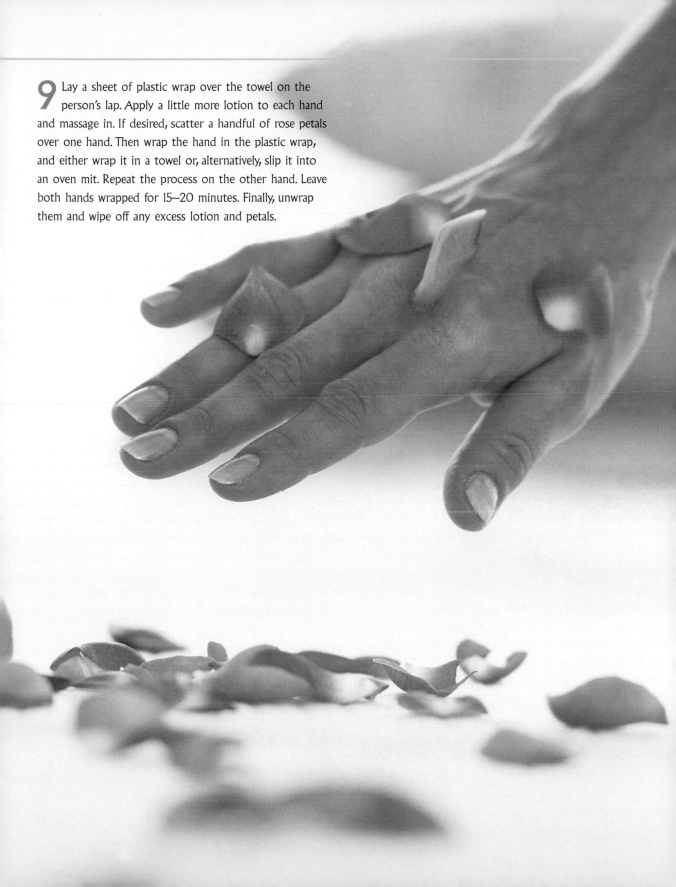

9 Lay a sheet of plastic wrap over the towel on the person's lap. Apply a little more lotion to each hand and massage in. If desired, scatter a handful of rose petals over one hand. Then wrap the hand in the plastic wrap, and either wrap it in a towel or, alternatively, slip it into an oven mit. Repeat the process on the other hand. Leave both hands wrapped for 15–20 minutes. Finally, unwrap them and wipe off any excess lotion and petals.

BANISHING CELLULITE

Cellulite occurs when toxins cause fat cells to swell and become trapped in the connective layer of tissue under the skin, resulting in a dimpled effect. Massage can help reduce the appearance of cellulite by boosting circulation, which helps to flush out toxins, and by improving the elasticity of the connective tissue. Cellulite appears most commonly on the thighs, buttocks, and upper arms. This massage can be easily adapted for any of those areas. Use a mixture of three parts moisturizing lotion to one part witch hazel.

REDUCING CELLULITE

Take the following steps to help reduce the appearance of cellulite:
• Drink 6–8 cups (1 1/2–2 liters) of water a day to help flush out toxins.
• Avoid caffeine and don't smoke.
• Body brush regularly in the bath or shower to boost blood flow to the skin.
• Exercise regularly, at least three times a week, to help boost circulation.

1 With alternate hands, perform brisk, rhythmic CUPPING all over the back of the thigh. The skin should redden slightly, an indication that blood flow to the area is stimulated. Repeat at least 10 times.

curve hands and keep fingers together when cupping

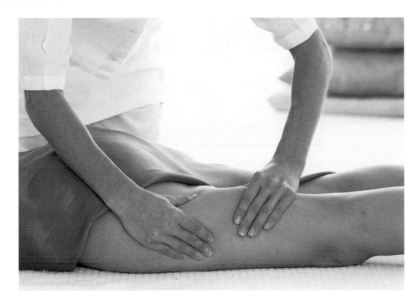

2 Perform TWO-HANDED KNEADING on the thigh by grasping and squeezing the flesh between the fingers and thumb of one hand, then pushing it toward the other hand to begin kneading. Repeat the process, applying firm pressure and kneading the flesh from hand to hand. Work methodically all over the area.

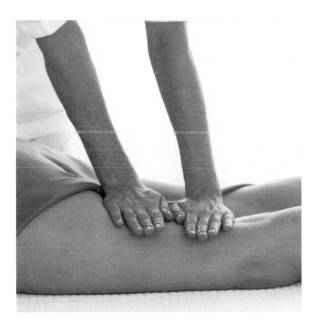

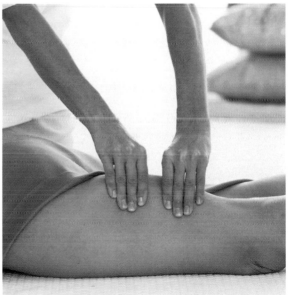

3 Perform the two stages of LIFTING: place both hands flat on the back of the thigh and, with fingers closed, apply pressure, leaning forward to increase the intensity.

4 Then grasp the flesh between the fingers and thumbs of both hands and pull upward, gently squeezing. Repeat the pressing and lifting action at least 6 times, taking care to avoid the back of the knee.

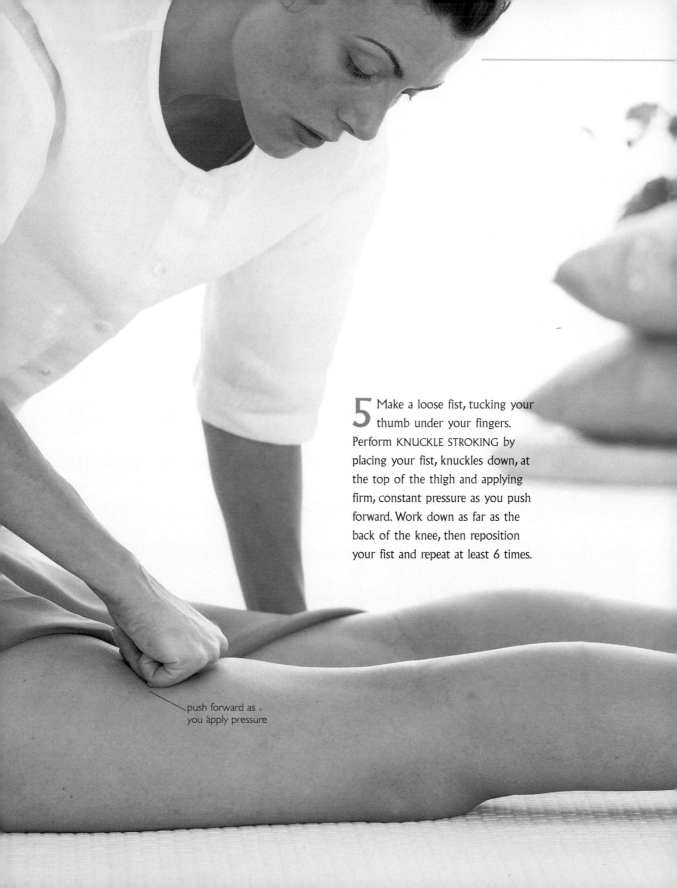

5 Make a loose fist, tucking your thumb under your fingers. Perform KNUCKLE STROKING by placing your fist, knuckles down, at the top of the thigh and applying firm, constant pressure as you push forward. Work down as far as the back of the knee, then reposition your fist and repeat at least 6 times.

push forward as you apply pressure

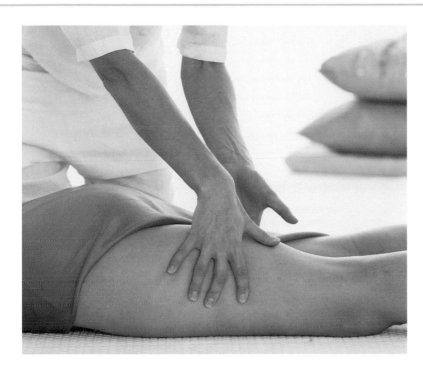

6 Splaying your fingers, place your hands on either side of the thigh. Perform SHAKING by pushing the thigh back and forth from one hand to the other.

SELF-MASSAGE FOR CELLULITE

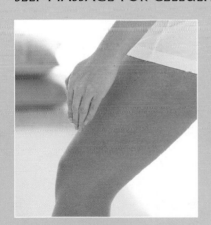

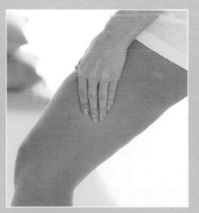

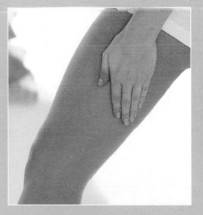

1 Perform CUPPING by tapping your cupped hand over the entire thigh area. Repeat at least 10 times.

2 Perform ONE-HANDED KNEADING by pushing and squeezing the flesh between your fingers and thumb, then releasing It. Work up and down the thigh. Repeat at least 10 times.

3 Place your hand flat against your thigh and shake it, sending vibrations through it. Shake for at least one minute.

BAREFOOT IN THE PARK

The height of decadence and one of the most popular treatments at my spa, this four-stage pampering routine is as luxurious as a facial, but it is meant for the feet. It consists of a soothing foot bath, a relaxing massage, and an exfoliating scrub. To finish, an enriching kiwi foot mask is applied. Use a little oil or lotion for the foot massage, and set aside at least 45 minutes to perform the entire treatment. Remember that you need a towel and two pieces of plastic wrap large enough to wrap the feet.

RELAXING FOOT BATHS

Try these alternative recipes for foot baths. Pour enough hot water to cover the feet into a bowl or foot bath.
• For puffy ankles and water retention, add a handful of fresh sage leaves and 3 drops of sage essential oil.
• For a cleansing effect that will leave feet feeling refreshed, add 2 tea bags of green tea or 4 tsp of green tea leaves.

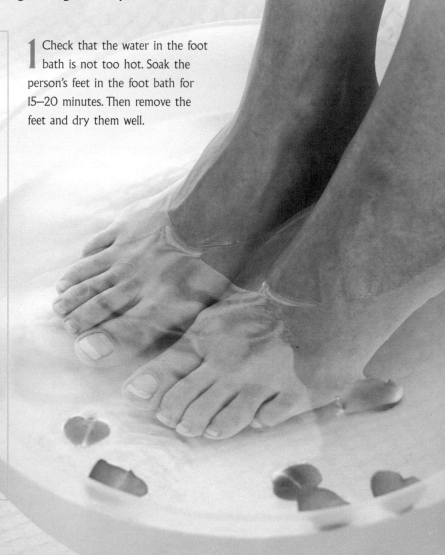

ROSE FOOT BATH

◆ enough hot water to cover feet in a foot bath or bowl (temperature guide: 1 cup boiling water to 3 cups cold water)

◆ a handful of fresh rose petals

◆ 1 tsp salt

◆ 3 drops rose essential oil

Mix all the ingredients together in a foot bath or bowl.

SALT RUB

◆ ¹/₄ cup (2oz) coarse sea salt

◆ enough grapeseed or sunflower oil to cover the salt

Mix all the ingredients in a bowl.

KIWI FOOT MASK

◆ 3 fresh kiwis, puréed in a food processor or mashed with a fork

◆ 3 tsp oil such as sweet almond, grapeseed, or sunflower

Mix all the ingredients in a bowl.

1 Check that the water in the foot bath is not too hot. Soak the person's feet in the foot bath for 15–20 minutes. Then remove the feet and dry them well.

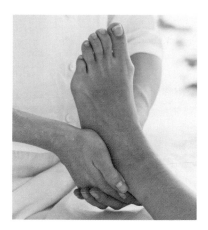

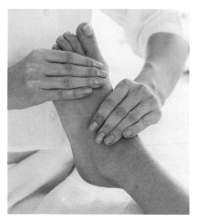

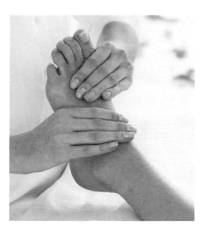

2 Interlock your fingers and cradle the heel of the foot in your hands. Apply pressure with the heels of your hands, holding for a count of 5, then slowly releasing. Repeat several times.

3 Grasp the foot, positioning one hand over the instep and the other slightly above it. Squeeze the foot between the fingers and thumb of each hand.

4 Keeping your fingers together, firmly pull and squeeze the foot. As one hand finishes the movement, begin pulling and squeezing with the other, as if pulling an endless length of toffee.

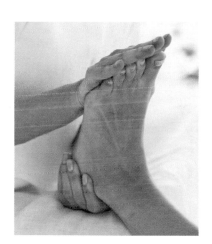

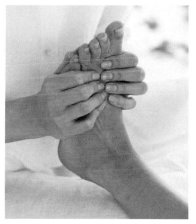

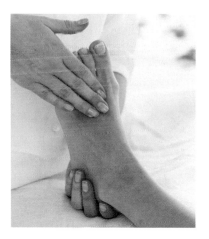

5 Support the heel of the foot in one hand and place your other hand, fingers up, on the ball of the foot. Push forward, gently stretching the foot, for a count of 5, then release for a count of 5. Repeat several times.

6 Grasp the foot with both hands, positioning your thumbs next to each other on the fleshy area below the toes. Perform THUMB FANNING, stretching the sole of the foot as you glide your thumbs outward. Repeat, working down the foot.

7 Support the heel of the foot in one hand. With the index and middle fingers of the other hand, trace between the tendons that run from the toes to the ankle, applying moderate pressure. Repeat several times.

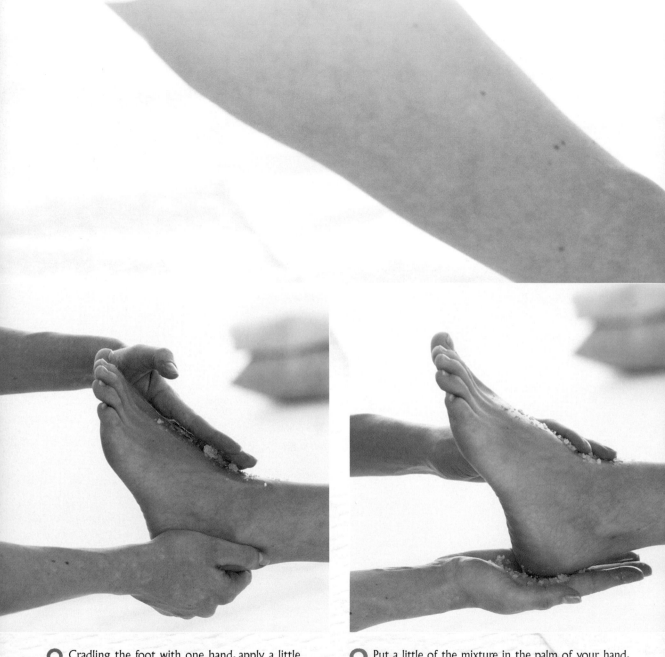

8 Cradling the foot with one hand, apply a little of the exfoliating salt and oil mixture to the top of the foot with the other. The skin here is quite delicate so apply the mixture gently, stroking rather than rubbing.

9 Put a little of the mixture in the palm of your hand, and apply it to the heel with a circular movement. Rub over hard or callused areas such as the backs of the heels and along the sides of the foot, varying the pressure and briskness of the strokes as necessary. Rinse and dry the foot. Repeat steps 2–9 on the other foot.

10 Lay a towel on the floor and on it place two pieces of plastic wrap or sheeting large enough to wrap each foot. Position the feet in the middle of the plastic wrap or sheeting and apply the moisturizing kiwi foot mask, covering the entire foot.

spread the mixture evenly over the feet

11 Wrap each foot in plastic wrap or sheeting, then fold the towel over to cover the feet entirely. Leave for 15 minutes, then unwrap, wipe off the mixture, and rinse the feet clean.

SEASONAL BODY SCRUB

Slough away dead skin cells to reveal smooth, healthy skin with a soothing exfoliating massage. Regular scrubbing and buffing helps eliminate dry scaly patches and gives the skin a warm glow. Choose a seasonal exfoliator from the selection below, and tailor this treatment to your needs. Concentrate on typically dry areas such as the feet, elbows, and knees, or massage the whole body. At the end of the treatment, rinse off the exfoliating mixture and apply a moisturizer of your choice.

EXFOLIATION TIPS

• Ideally, try to exfoliate at least once every two weeks.
• Always exfoliate before applying any self-tanning product—focus in particular on the elbows, knees, and any hard or callused areas on the feet.
• **Do not** exfoliate areas with severe acne as this may cause scarring.

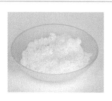

WINTER EXFOLIATOR

Central heating dries out the skin. Use this mixture to nourish parched skin and to help eliminate rough patches.

◆ ¹/₂ cup (125g) sea salt
◆ ¹/₂ cup (125ml) oil such as sweet almond, grapeseed, or sunflower
◆ 6 drops peppermint essential oil

Mix all the ingredients together in a bowl.

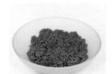

SPRING EXFOLIATOR

This gentle orange-scented scrub loosens dead skin cells and revitalizes to give skin a soft, healthy glow.

◆ ¹/₂ cup (125g) poppy seeds
◆ ¹/₂ cup (125ml) oil such as sweet almond, grapeseed, or sunflower
◆ 5 drops orange essential oil

Mix all the ingredients together in a bowl.

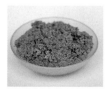

SUMMER EXFOLIATOR

The active enzyme in strawberries cleanses and brightens the skin, while oatmeal acts as a gentle buffing agent.

◆ 1 cup (250g) oatmeal
◆ 12 ripe strawberries or 3 kiwis, mashed or puréed
◆ a little water

Mix the oatmeal and mashed fruit together in a bowl. Stir in water as necessary until the mixture is the consistency of thick paste.

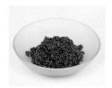

FALL EXFOLIATOR

Powdered walnut shell polishes and refines the skin. Before grinding, break shells into smaller pieces with a hammer.

◆ 3 tbsp powdered walnut shell, or 10 walnut shells finely ground in a coffee grinder
◆ ¹/₄ cup (75ml) oil such as sweet almond, grapeseed, or sunflower
◆ 5 drops cinnamon essential oil

Mix all the ingredients together in a bowl.

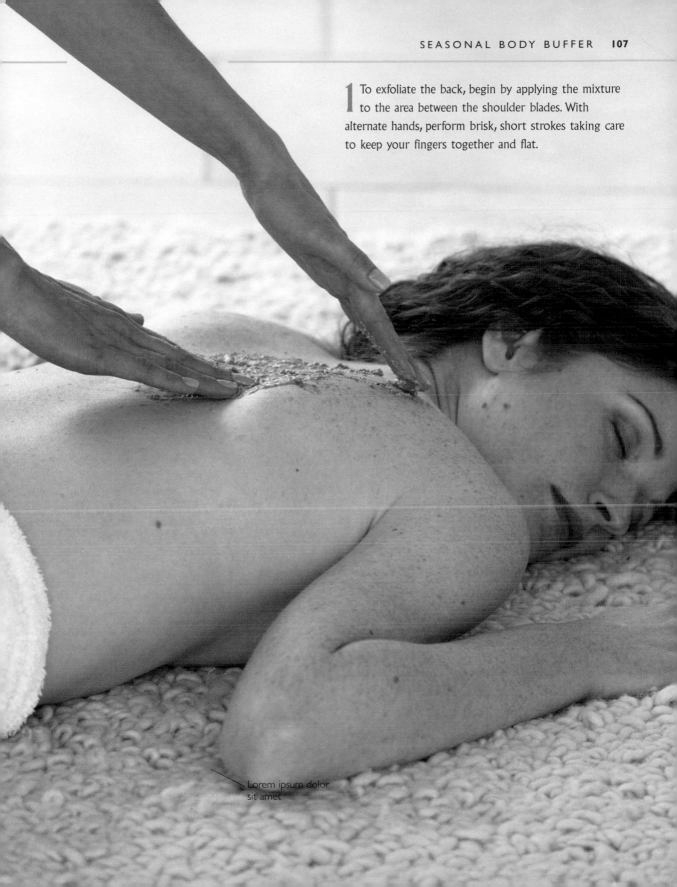

1 To exfoliate the back, begin by applying the mixture to the area between the shoulder blades. With alternate hands, perform brisk, short strokes taking care to keep your fingers together and flat.

Lorem ipsum dolor sit amet

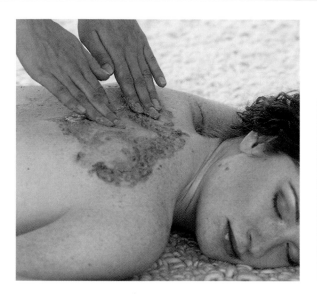

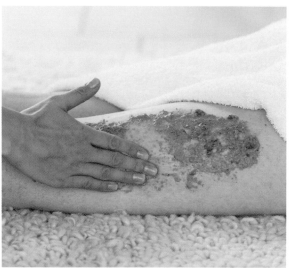

2 Use four fingers and work across the back from one shoulder to the other, performing small circular movements while applying moderate pressure. If desired, use this technique to cover the whole back.

3 To exfoliate the leg, apply a little of the mixture to the back of the thigh and perform LIGHT LONG STROKING with one hand. Spread the mixture evenly over the entire leg, applying moderate pressure as you stroke.

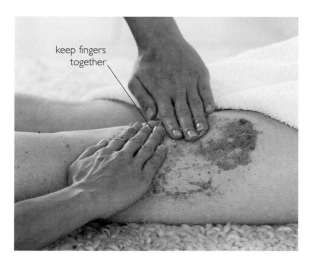

keep fingers together

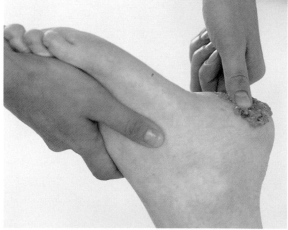

4 Place one hand slightly above the other on the leg with fingers flat and pointing inward. Perform V-FORMATION STROKING, sliding your hands outward, then in again. Repeat, moving up and down the leg, then perform steps 3 and 4 on the other leg.

5 To exfoliate the foot, support it with one hand as you apply a little of the mixture to the heel with the other. Work around the entire heel area, applying THUMB PRESSURE in small circular movements.

6 Apply a little more of the mixture to the heel if necessary. Cup your hand over the heel and apply pressure as you circle your palm around it. Repeat several times.

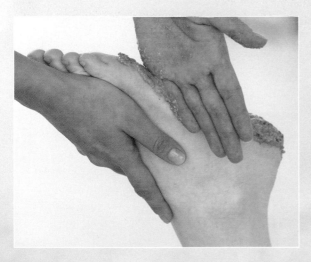

7 Still supporting the foot with one hand, use your other hand to perform SAWING. Work along the edges of the foot using brisk strokes performed with the side of your hand. Then repeat steps 5–7 to exfoliate the other foot.

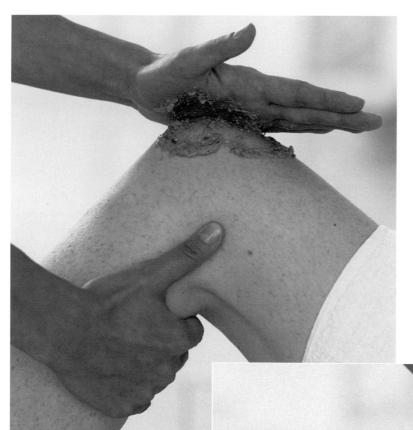

8 To exfoliate the knee, bend the leg and hold it steady with one hand as you apply a little of the mixture with the palm of your other hand. Apply pressure with a circular movement as if rolling a ball under your hand.

9 Work around the knee cap applying circular thumb pressure. Apply more exfoliating mixture as necessary.

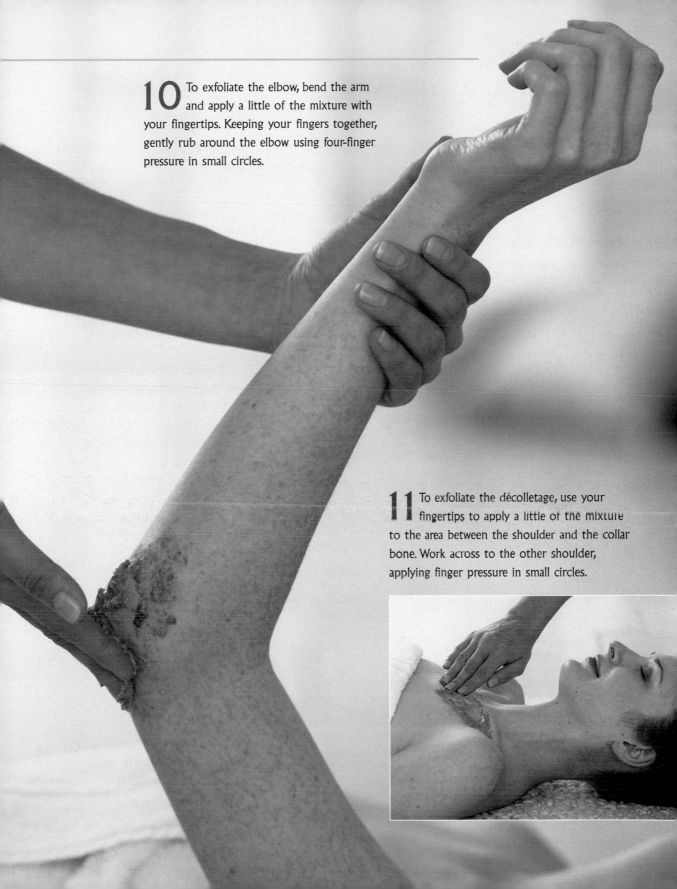

10 To exfoliate the elbow, bend the arm and apply a little of the mixture with your fingertips. Keeping your fingers together, gently rub around the elbow using four-finger pressure in small circles.

11 To exfoliate the décolletage, use your fingertips to apply a little of the mixture to the area between the shoulder and the collar bone. Work across to the other shoulder, applying finger pressure in small circles.

PAPAYA WRAP

This intensive moisturizing treatment rehydrates and nourishes the skin. Papain, the enzyme in papaya, breaks down dead skin cells, allowing the oil in the wrap mixture to penetrate more effectively to help restore the skin's natural moisture balance. Try substituting mango or pineapple for the papaya—all of these exotic fruits contain valuable natural enzymes that leave the skin soft and glowing. Lie back, breathe in the fruit-scented aromas, and imagine a warm tropical paradise.

HOW TO WRAP

Spread a blanket on the floor and layer one more blanket and a towel on top. Spread a plastic sheet or a plastic table cloth (shiny side up) over the towel. Lie the person down and apply the wrap mixture. Fold the top edge of the plastic over to prevent leakage, then wrap by folding first the plastic over the person, then the layers of towel and blankets.

PAPAYA WRAP MIXTURE

- 1 large papaya, seeded and mashed with a fork or puréed, or 1 large mango, pit removed, finely chopped or puréed, or 1 small pineapple, peeled and finely chopped or puréed
- 1/4 cup (75ml) oil such as sweet almond, grapeseed, or cold-pressed sunflower

Mix the ingredients together in a bowl.

Also needed:

- 2 blankets and 1 towel
- plastic sheet or tablecloth
- extra towels for draping over the person during the treatment and for wiping away excess mixture

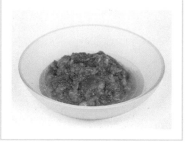

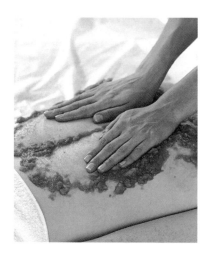

1 Lie the person face down on the plastic sheeting with his or her head above the plastic. Using the PAINTING stroke, apply half of the wrap mixture to the back of the body, starting on the back. Place your hands flat on the body and use FANNING to spread the mixture over the body and backs of the arms and legs.

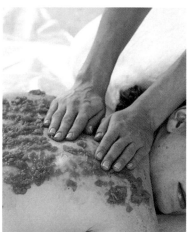

2 Place your hands flat on the back and, keeping your fingers together, perform gentle FULL-HAND COMPRESSIONS to spread the mixture evenly and to press it against the skin. Start on the back, then move to the backs of the legs and the arms. Do not perform compressions on the backs of the knees or elbows.

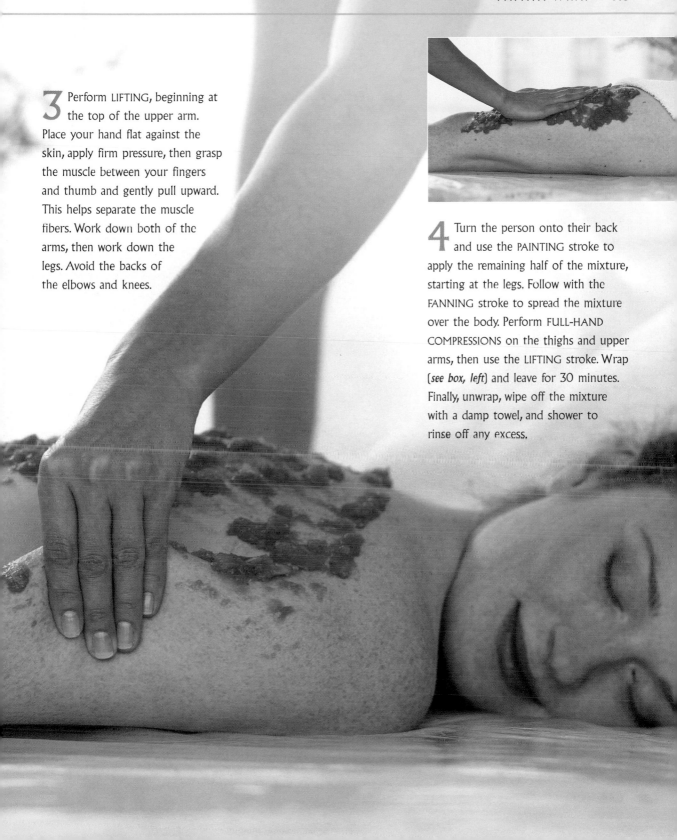

3 Perform LIFTING, beginning at the top of the upper arm. Place your hand flat against the skin, apply firm pressure, then grasp the muscle between your fingers and thumb and gently pull upward. This helps separate the muscle fibers. Work down both of the arms, then work down the legs. Avoid the backs of the elbows and knees.

4 Turn the person onto their back and use the PAINTING stroke to apply the remaining half of the mixture, starting at the legs. Follow with the FANNING stroke to spread the mixture over the body. Perform FULL-HAND COMPRESSIONS on the thighs and upper arms, then use the LIFTING stroke. Wrap (*see box, left*) and leave for 30 minutes. Finally, unwrap, wipe off the mixture with a damp towel, and shower to rinse off any excess.

GINGER WRAP

This two-stage treatment consists of a brisk "surface" massage with cinnamon oil to help boost blood flow to the skin followed by a stimulating ginger-infused wrap. Body heat generated by the swaddling process opens the pores and encourages optimum absorption of the wrap mixture. Before the treatment, prepare for the wrap by laying down blankets and plastic sheeting (*see box, p.112*). Remember to fold over the top edge of the plastic sheeting before wrapping to prevent the ginger mixture from leaking out.

BOOSTING CIRCULATION

This ginger wrap invigorates and can temporarily boost circulation; you might also try the following:
• To boost circulation, stand up, raise your arms above your head, and shake your hands for 10–15 seconds. Then relax your arms by your sides.
• Take regular hot baths to help improve circulation.

CINNAMON MASSAGE OIL

Add 5 drops of cinnamon essential oil to 2 tsp (10ml) almond oil.

GINGER WRAP MIXTURE

• 1 large fresh piece of ginger, at least 6in (15cm), finely grated by hand or in a food processor
• ½ cup (125ml) oil such as sweet almond, grapeseed, or sunflower

Mix the ingredients together in a bowl.

Also needed:
• 2 blankets and 1 towel
• plastic sheet or tablecloth
• extra towels for draping over the person during the treatment and for wiping away excess mixture

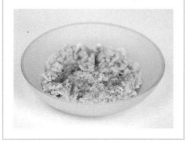

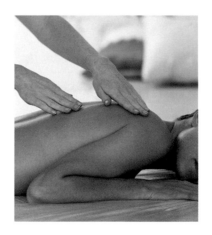

1 Rub a little cinnamon oil into your hands. With the person lying on his or her front, begin with light, brisk HAND-OVER-HAND STROKING on the back. As you finish a stroke and lift one hand off the body, begin stroking upward with the other. Then place your hands flat on the upper back and perform FANNING over the sides of the torso to the lower back.

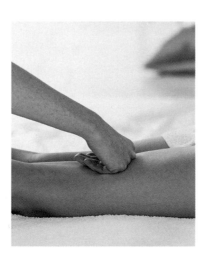

2 Move to the feet, and with one hand holding the foot, perform KNUCKLE STROKING up the back of the calf, applying firm pressure. Lighten the pressure over the backs of the knees. Repeat on the other leg, then turn the person over and work up one leg and then the other using brisk, light HAND-OVER-HAND STROKING.

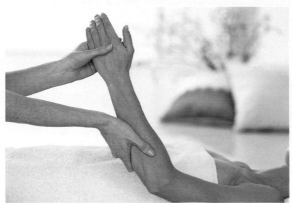

3 Holding the person's hand in one hand, perform ONE-HANDED KNEADING up the entire arm, firmly grasping and squeezing the flesh. Then knead up the other arm. Next, sit the person up and apply the ginger wrap mixture to the back before lying them down again.

4 Apply the ginger mixture to the legs, bending the knee to reach under the leg. Then apply the mixture to the feet, arms, and abdomen using a combination of PAINTING and FANNING, and finally wrap the person (*see box, p.112*). Leave to rest undisturbed for at least 30 minutes, then unwrap, wipe off the mixture with a damp towel, and shower.

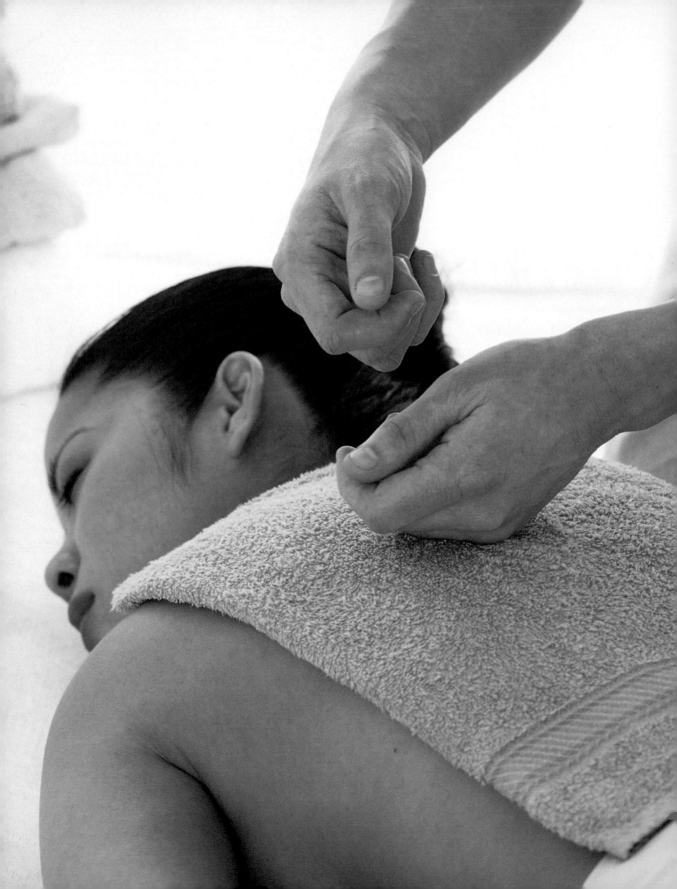

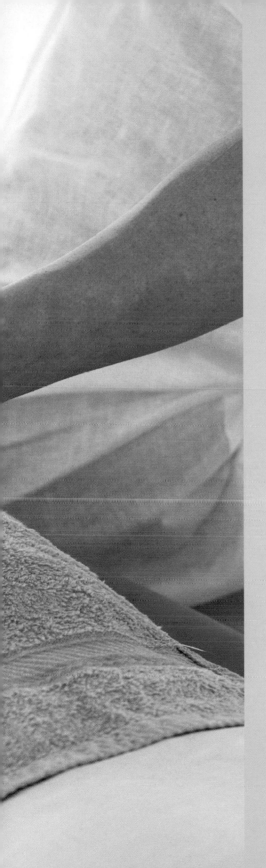

MASSAGE FOR HEALTH

With tension and stress at the root of so

many of our health problems, therapeutic

massage can play an essential role in

improving and maintaining our health and

well-being. The routines that follow not

only induce relaxation, they teach you

how to use massage to ease the pain of

headaches, stress knots, and lower back

discomfort. There is also a routine to

speed muscle recovery time after sports.

WORKING OUT KNOTS

Stress knots tend to form in the rhomboids (*see pp.8–9*), the muscles that run from the spine to the shoulder blade. They feel like small, hard pebbles and can be caused by stress or activities such as typing or carrying a heavy shoulder bag. Here, the knot is located between the person's spine and right shoulder blade. Use oil for this massage, and apply hard pressure, but not enough to cause pain. Work on each knot until you feel it breaking down. Prepare a hot towel (*see p.122*) before you begin.

TREATING STRESS KNOTS
• Add a cup of Epsom salts to a hot bath. Soak in the bath to help ease the pain of a stressed, knotted muscle.
• Try rolling a tennis ball around over the knot to help break it down.
• If there are several knots, finish working on one before you move on to the next.
• Try performing the back massage on pages 48–51 before this routine.

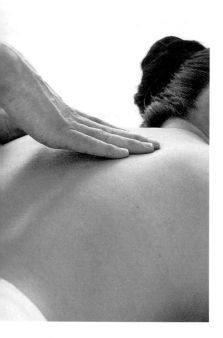 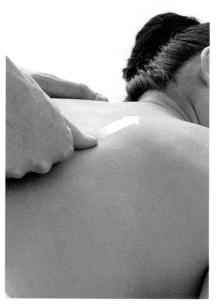 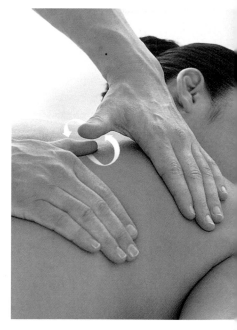

1 Begin by performing LIGHT LONG STROKING upward over the affected area. Repeat several times, working across as well as along the muscle as you gradually increase the pressure to perform DEEP LONG STROKING.

2 Focusing on the entire area between the spine and the shoulder blade, perform THUMB STRIPPING, working up the muscles along the right side of the spine. Repeat several times, applying constant, firm pressure.

3 Then work along the muscles at the side of the spine, performing THUMB-OVER-THUMB STROKING across the muscle fibers.

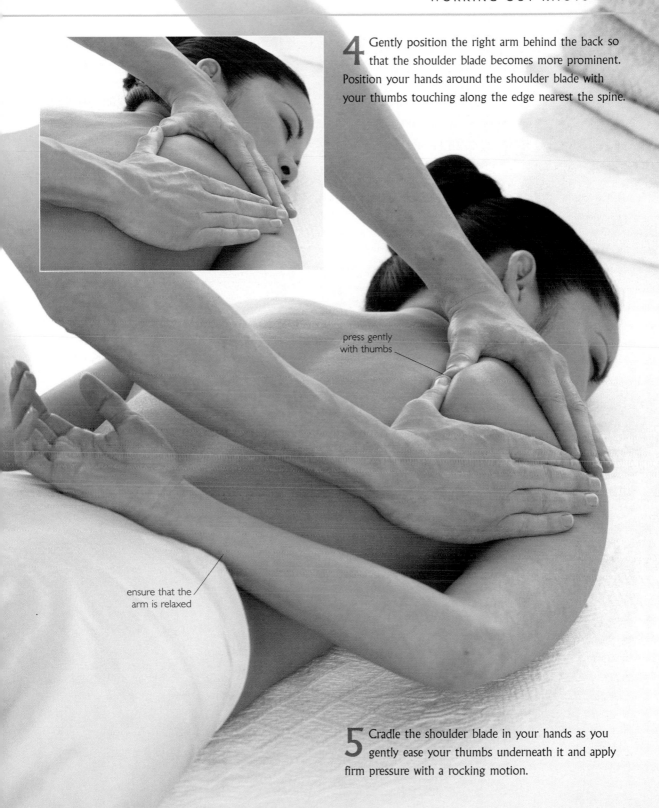

4 Gently position the right arm behind the back so that the shoulder blade becomes more prominent. Position your hands around the shoulder blade with your thumbs touching along the edge nearest the spine.

press gently
with thumbs

ensure that the
arm is relaxed

5 Cradle the shoulder blade in your hands as you gently ease your thumbs underneath it and apply firm pressure with a rocking motion.

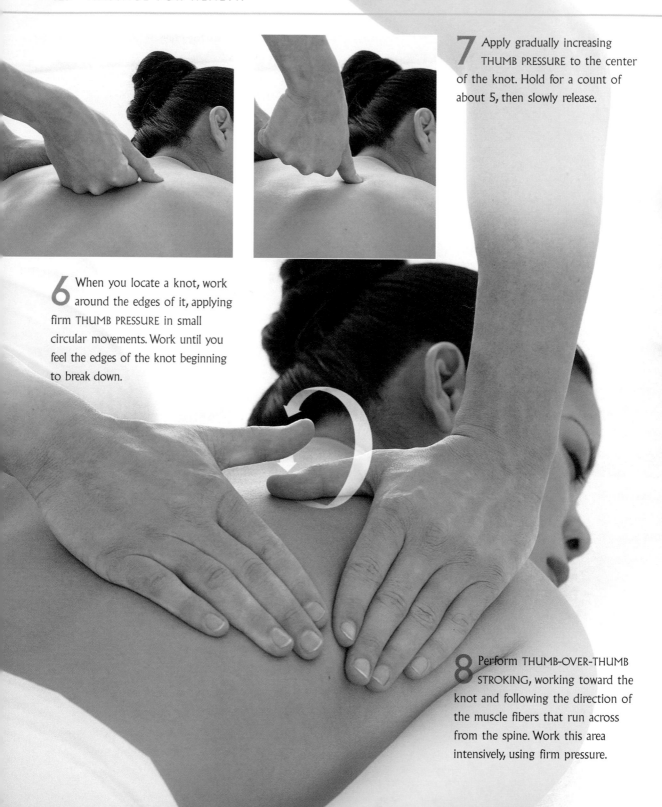

7 Apply gradually increasing THUMB PRESSURE to the center of the knot. Hold for a count of about 5, then slowly release.

6 When you locate a knot, work around the edges of it, applying firm THUMB PRESSURE in small circular movements. Work until you feel the edges of the knot beginning to break down.

8 Perform THUMB-OVER-THUMB STROKING, working toward the knot and following the direction of the muscle fibers that run across from the spine. Work this area intensively, using firm pressure.

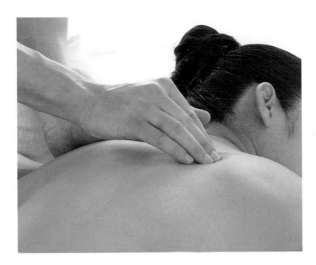

9 Place your fingertips together on the knotted area and apply firm pressure as you simultaneously shake your fingers to create vibration. Continue for about 15–20 seconds. Repeat as necessary until you feel the knot beginning to break down.

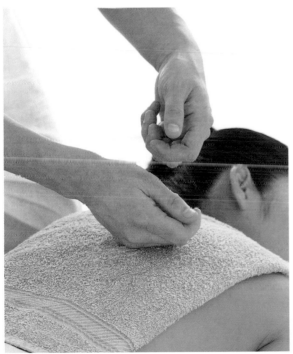

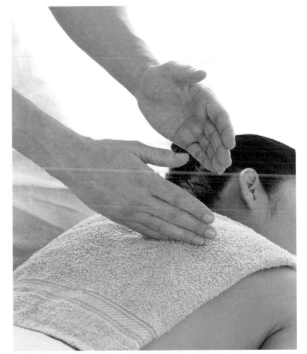

10 Place a hot towel over the back to help soften the knot and soothe and relax the muscle. Perform PUMMELING with firm pressure over the knot, taking care not to pummel directly on the spine.

11 Finish by performing HACKING over the affected area, varying both the pace and the pressure as necessary. Remove the towel, and finish by performing LIGHT LONG STROKING over the area.

SPORTS MASSAGE

Performed before exercise, a good sports massage prepares the muscles for action by stimulating blood flow to them, which helps to minimize aches, soreness, and cramps, and can even prevent injury. Post-exercise, this brisk massage will ease tired muscles while also having an invigorating effect. Try massaging with half a cup of witch hazel mixed with 5 drops of eucalyptus essential oil rather than just oil. Tight muscles can be loosened by applying a hot towel prior to massage (*see box*).

PREPARING A HOT TOWEL

Prepare a hot towel by dampening it, rolling it up, and placing it in the microwave for 2–3 minutes. Unroll and apply to the affected area when the towel has stopped steaming. Alternatively, soak the towel in 3 cups cold water and 1 cup boiling water, wring out, and apply.

Do not massage swollen, painful, or injured areas.

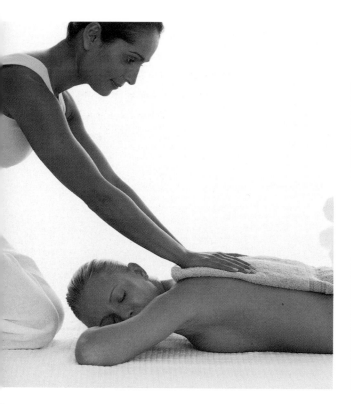

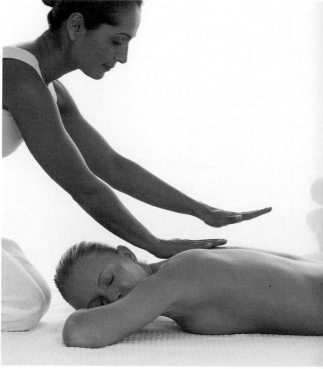

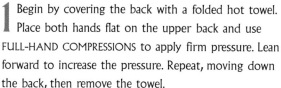

1 Begin by covering the back with a folded hot towel. Place both hands flat on the upper back and use FULL-HAND COMPRESSIONS to apply firm pressure. Lean forward to increase the pressure. Repeat, moving down the back, then remove the towel.

2 Perform brisk, short strokes between the shoulder blades, maintaining a rhythmic pace. This stimulates blood flow to the muscles in this area, increasing mobility in the neck and shoulders.

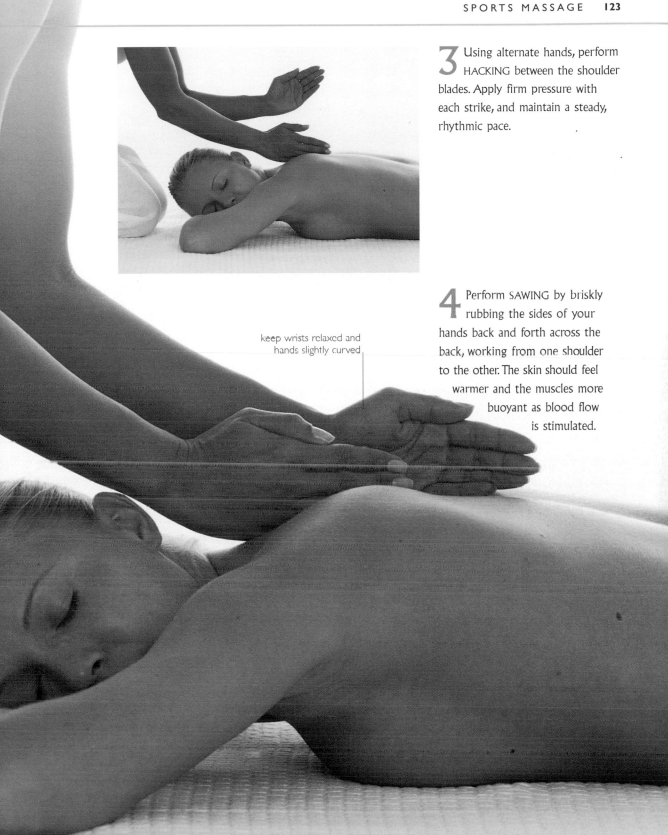

3 Using alternate hands, perform HACKING between the shoulder blades. Apply firm pressure with each strike, and maintain a steady, rhythmic pace.

keep wrists relaxed and hands slightly curved

4 Perform SAWING by briskly rubbing the sides of your hands back and forth across the back, working from one shoulder to the other. The skin should feel warmer and the muscles more buoyant as blood flow is stimulated.

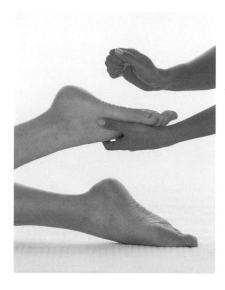

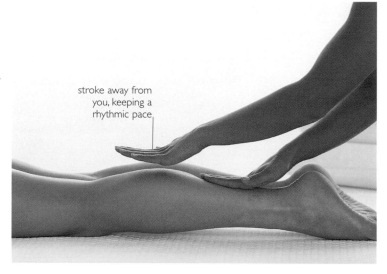

stroke away from
you, keeping a
rhythmic pace

5 Move to the feet. Hold a foot in one hand. With your other hand make a loose fist and tap it rhythmically against the sole of the foot. Repeat on the other foot.

6 Move to the legs and perform brisk HAND-OVER-HAND STROKING, working up the entire leg and including the buttocks. Work up the leg at least 3 times, taking care to keep the strokes short and rhythmic and remembering to keep your fingers together.

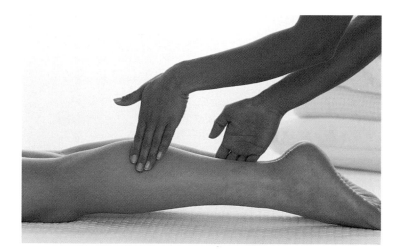

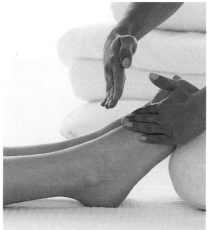

7 Place one hand on one side of the leg at the ankle and the other on the other side a little further up on the calf. Perform ROCKING, pushing the leg with one hand and catching it with the other. Use enough force to move the leg, but control the movement. Repeat, moving up the leg. Then repeat steps 6 and 7 on the other leg.

8 Turn the person over and use alternate hands to stroke toward you from the ankle to the toes. Maintain a rhythmic pace and a firm pressure. Repeat several times.

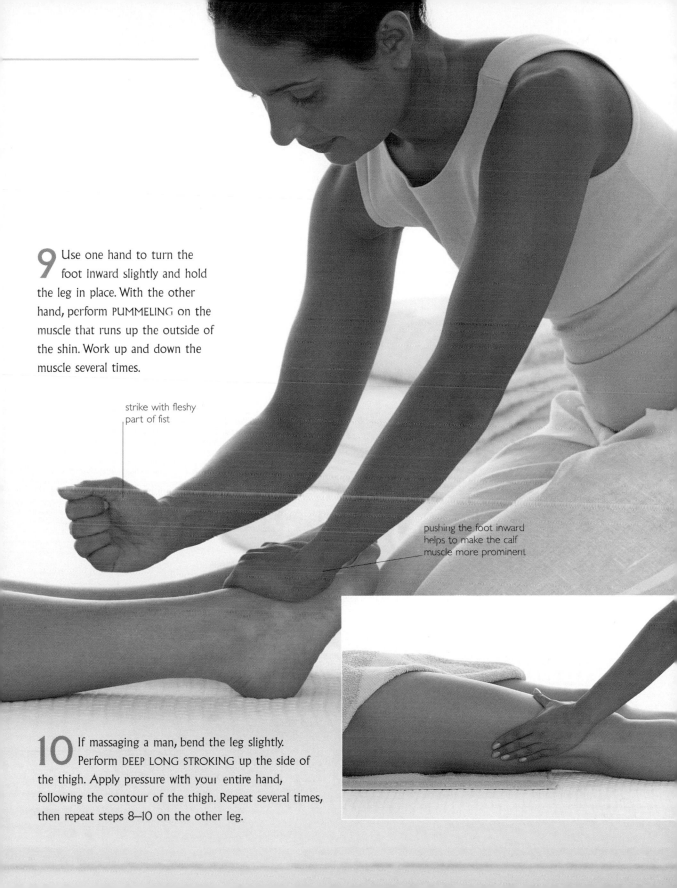

9 Use one hand to turn the foot inward slightly and hold the leg in place. With the other hand, perform PUMMELING on the muscle that runs up the outside of the shin. Work up and down the muscle several times.

strike with fleshy part of fist

pushing the foot inward helps to make the calf muscle more prominent

10 If massaging a man, bend the leg slightly. Perform DEEP LONG STROKING up the side of the thigh. Apply pressure with your entire hand, following the contour of the thigh. Repeat several times, then repeat steps 8–10 on the other leg.

11 To massage the abdominal muscles safely, reach over and place your right hand flat against the side of the abdomen. Forming your hand to the contour of the body, firmly pull your right hand toward you, sliding it over the top of the abdomen. As you do this, slide your left hand away from you over the abdomen so that both hands swap position.

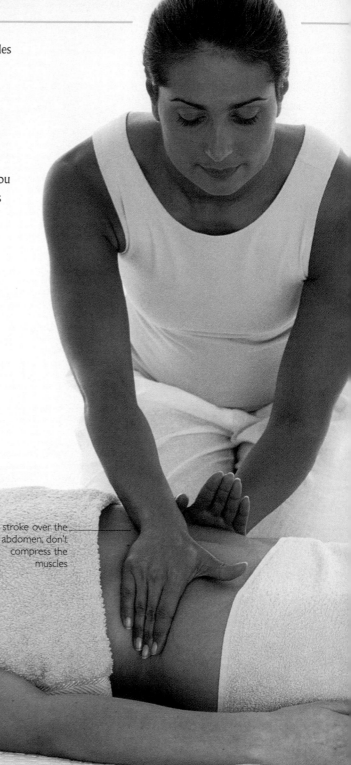

stroke over the abdomen; don't compress the muscles

12 Then repeat the movement, pulling with your left hand as you slide your right hand over the abdomen. Repeat the whole movement at least 3 times.

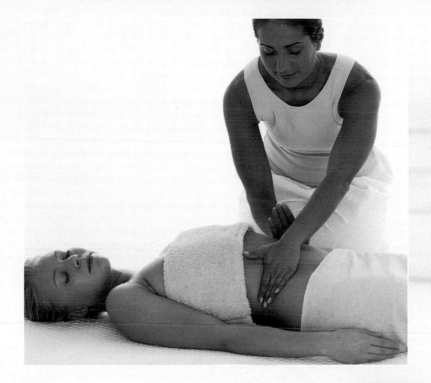

13 Perform ONE-HANDED KNEADING up the arm to the shoulder, avoiding the inside of the elbow. Repeat, then replace the arm by the side of the body. Finish the massage by kneading the other arm.

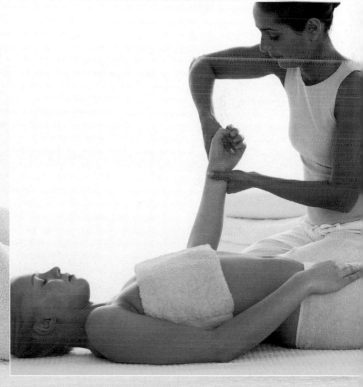

LYMPHATIC CLEANSING

The lymphatic system is one of the body's garbage disposal systems; it filters waste matter and bacteria from the blood. Lymph fluid circulates through the system, relying on breathing and muscle movement to flow, but massage also stimulates it. Use no oil or lotion for this massage, and apply very light pressure; the intention is to "sweep" toxins toward the lymph nodes in the neck, armpits, elbows, groin, and knees. The treatment consists of three basic strokes, all performed in the direction of the lymph nodes.

WHEN TO CLEANSE?

• For best results, this massage should be performed regularly, ideally about once a week. I also recommend this massage as an effective hangover remedy.

• Symptoms of a sluggish lymphatic system can include: poor immune function, blotchiness, blemishes, cellulite, bad breath, and body odor. Regular massage may reduce these symptoms.

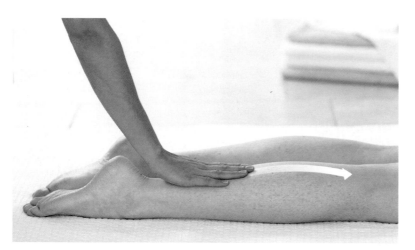

1 Begin with the person lying on his or her front. Start at the ankle, and perform gentle LIGHT LONG STROKING in the direction of the back of the knee. Take care to keep your fingers together and your hand flat. Repeat 3 times.

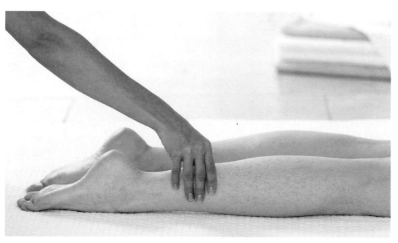

2 Place your hand flat against the ankle and perform LIFTING: apply firm pressure for 3–4 seconds, then grasp the flesh and squeeze gently as you pull upward. Move up the calf, repeating the pressing and pulling action. At the back of the knee, trail your fingers back down to the ankle and repeat LIFTING, working up the leg 2 more times.

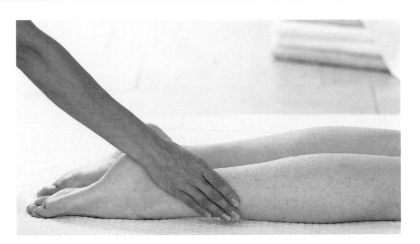

3 Start at the ankle again and perform an adapted version of ONE-HANDED KNEADING: begin by squeezing and pulling the flesh between your thumb and fingers.

4 Rather than releasing the flesh, slide your fingers forward and flick your hand away from the body as if to "sweep" toxins up the leg. Repeat the entire movement, working up to the back of the knee. Then trail your fingers back to the ankle and knead up the leg 2 more times.

control the flicking action with your wrist

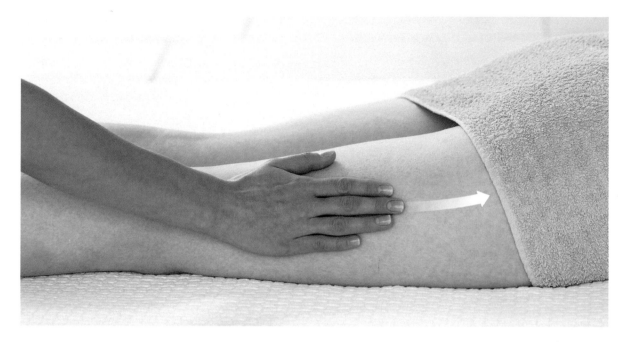

5 Move to the back of the thigh and repeat steps 1–4, starting with LIGHT LONG STROKING, then performing LIFTING and KNEADING. Work from the back of the knee to the buttock 3 times for each stroke. Then repeat the entire process on the other leg.

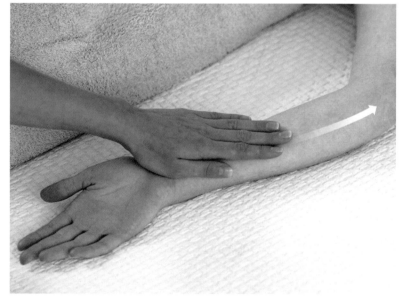

6 Move to the arm, and bend it slightly so that the palm faces upward and the arm is flat. Repeat steps 1–4 on the underside of the lower arm, working up the arm to the elbow 3 times for each stroke. Then move up the arm and repeat steps 1–4 on the underside of the upper arm, working from the inside of the elbow to the shoulder. Then repeat the entire process on the other arm.

7 Turn the person over onto his or her back and place a folded towel or small pillow under the neck for comfort. Starting at the ankle, work up toward the knee, performing LIGHT LONG STROKING, LIFTING, and KNEADING 3 times each. Repeat this sequence of strokes 3 times each to the calf and thigh of the other leg and then to both the lower and upper parts of the arms.

keep long strokes light and rhythmic

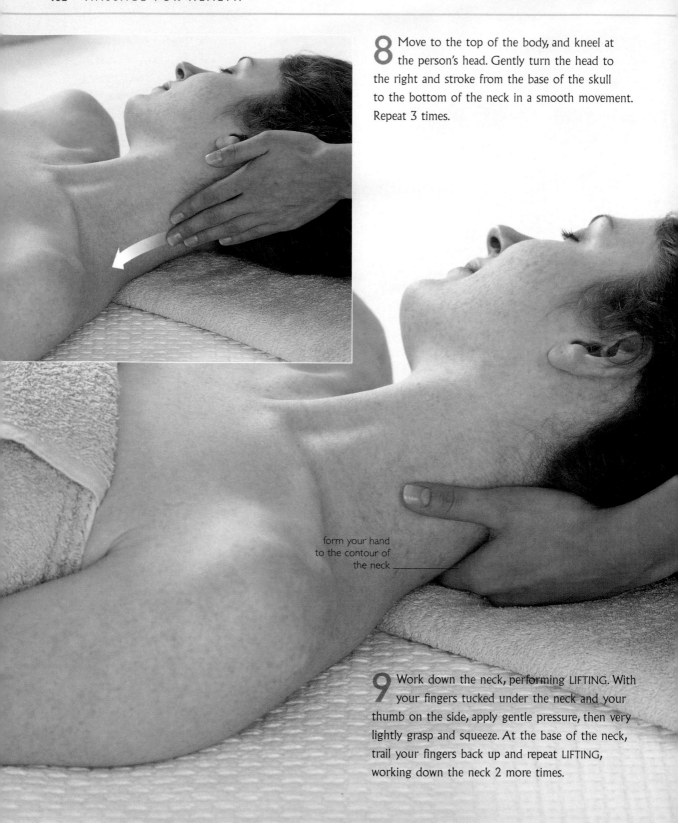

8 Move to the top of the body, and kneel at the person's head. Gently turn the head to the right and stroke from the base of the skull to the bottom of the neck in a smooth movement. Repeat 3 times.

form your hand to the contour of the neck _____

9 Work down the neck, performing LIFTING. With your fingers tucked under the neck and your thumb on the side, apply gentle pressure, then very lightly grasp and squeeze. At the base of the neck, trail your fingers back up and repeat LIFTING, working down the neck 2 more times.

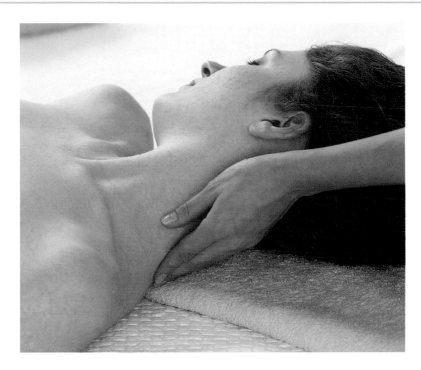

10 Finally, perform a two-step sweeping and flicking action down the neck. Begin by gliding your fingers down the back of the neck.

11 Flick your hand upward as if to brush away toxins. Repeat this sweeping and flicking stroke, working down to the base of the neck. Then trail your fingers back up to the base of the skull and work down the neck 2 more times. Finish by performing several sweeping long strokes down the neck. Then turn the head to the left and repeat steps 8–11 on the right side of the neck. Finish by gently turning the head to the center.

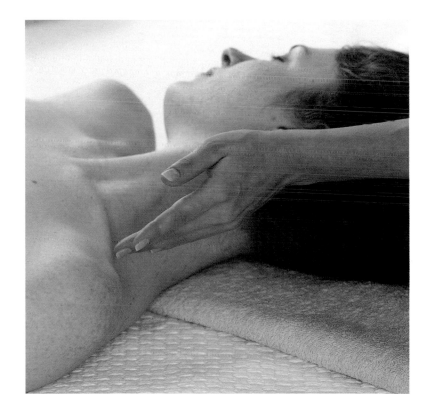

MELT AWAY HEADACHES

Headaches can be caused by factors such as muscle tension, allergic reaction, hormones, squinting, and sinus problems, but the most common cause is stress. With today's hectic schedules, it's not surprising that 90 percent of North American adults have experienced a tension headache. Before you begin, make an ice pack by wrapping a few ice cubes in a towel. The coolness eases the pain by causing swollen blood vessels that may be pressing against sensitive nerves to contract. No oil or lotion is required.

SELF-HELP FOR HEADACHES

• Sensitivity to certain foods and additives can cause headaches. Try eliminating the following from your diet and then gradually re-introducing them: alcohol, aspartame, caffeine, chocolate, and monosodium glutamate (MSG).

• Try deep breathing into a paper bag. Inhaling air containing increased levels of carbon dioxide helps to relax you.

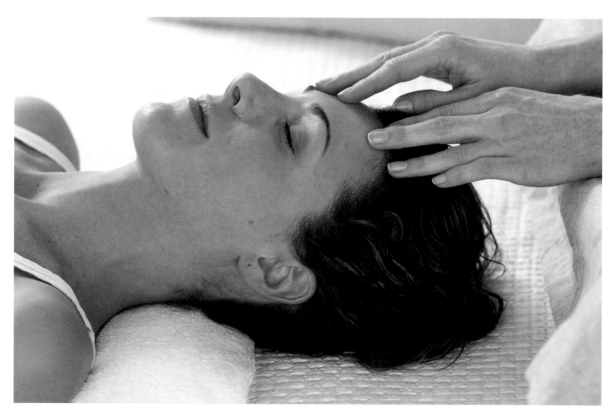

1 Place the ice pack under the neck. Begin by performing gentle, rhythmic strokes with alternate hands, sweeping up the forehead from the eyebrows to the hairline.

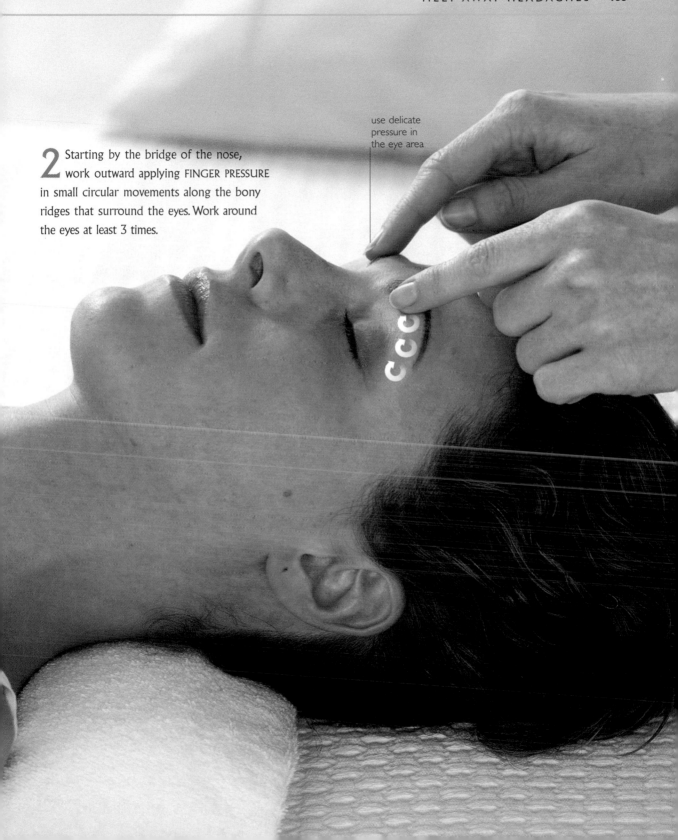

2 Starting by the bridge of the nose, work outward applying FINGER PRESSURE in small circular movements along the bony ridges that surround the eyes. Work around the eyes at least 3 times.

use delicate pressure in the eye area

3 Move the ice pack from under the neck and place it on the upper chest, at the bottom of the neck. Grasp the meaty flesh between the shoulders and neck (on both sides of the head) and gently pull for a count of 5, then slowly release. Repeat 3 times.

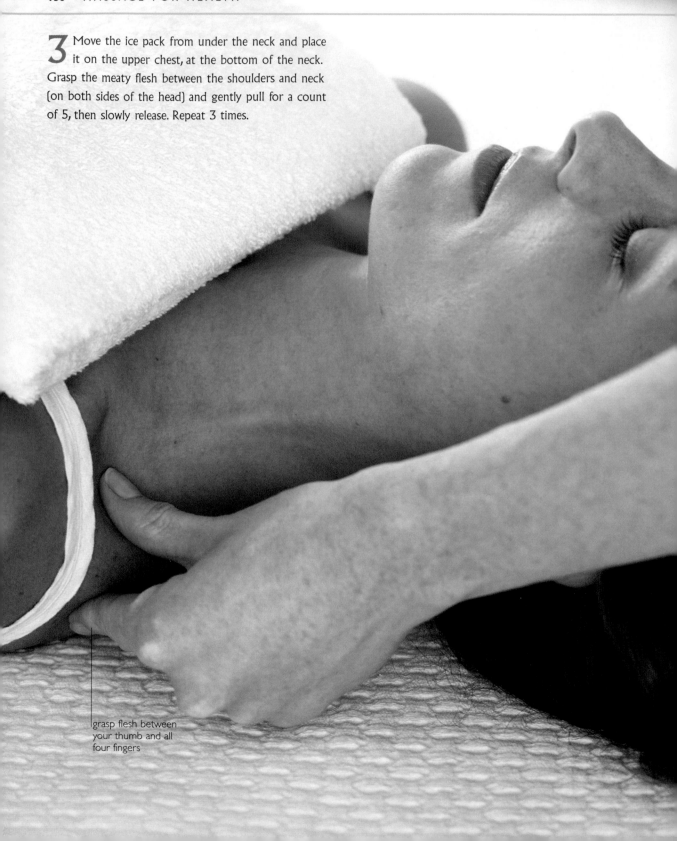

grasp flesh between
your thumb and all
four fingers

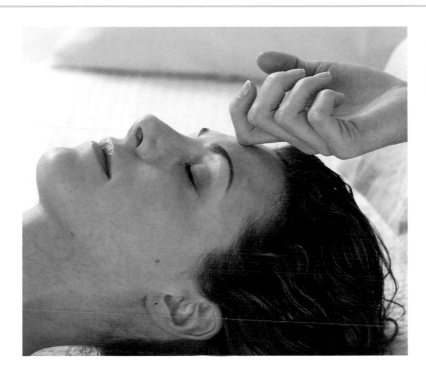

4 Use the knuckle of your index finger to tap the forehead gently. Lightly and rhythmically strike the center of the forehead 10 times.

SELF-MASSAGE FOR HEADACHES

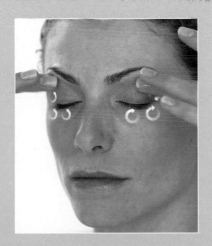

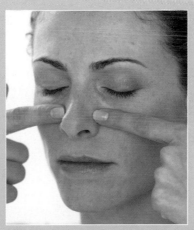

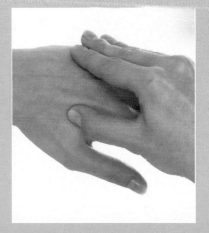

1 Use your middle fingers to work around the bony edges of the eye sockets applying FINGER PRESSURE in small circular patterns. Work around the eye at least 3 times.

2 Apply FINGER PRESSURE to the acupressure points on either side of the nostrils. Gradually increase pressure for a count of 5, then release for a count of 5.

3 Apply gradually increasing THUMB PRESSURE to the acupressure point at the base of your index finger. Hold for a count of 5, then slowly release. This may feel achy.

LOWER BACK PAIN RELIEF

Most people suffer from lower back pain at one time or another in their life. A common cause is weak abdominal muscles, which force the back to work harder to keep the body upright. Before you begin the massage, check the temperature of the area. If it feels hot, the muscles are inflamed and you should keep the pressure light. Otherwise use firm pressure, but check with the person that it is comfortable. Applying a hot towel (*see box, p.122*) helps to relax the muscles. Use oil or lotion for this massage.

PREVENTING BACK PAIN

• Exercise regularly and maintain a healthy weight; do exercises such as sit-ups that strengthen your abdominals.
• Minimize stress to the lower back by always bending your knees when lifting and moving objects.

Never massage individuals with acute back pain or with pain that shoots down the leg. Refer them to a doctor.

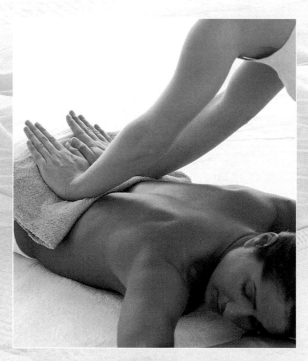

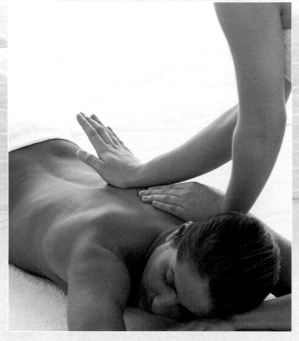

1 Place a hot towel on the lower back and, kneeling at the person's head, perform HEEL-OF-HAND COMPRESSIONS through the towel. Lean forward and apply firm pressure combined with shaking to loosen and relax the muscles. Move around the area, applying this technique for at least one minute, then remove the towel.

2 Place one hand on the upper back to hold the skin steady, and perform HEEL-OF-HAND STROKING with the other hand. Glide down as far as the buttocks, leaning forward to apply firm pressure. Repeat several times. Lighten pressure over the kidneys (in the small of the back) and avoid stroking directly on the spine.

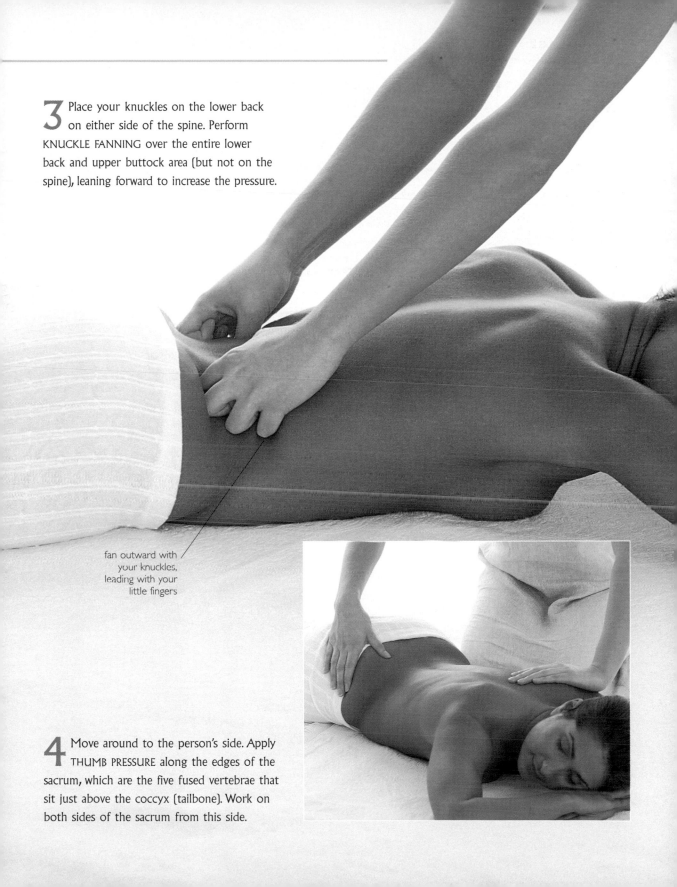

3 Place your knuckles on the lower back on either side of the spine. Perform KNUCKLE FANNING over the entire lower back and upper buttock area (but not on the spine), leaning forward to increase the pressure.

fan outward with your knuckles, leading with your little fingers

4 Move around to the person's side. Apply THUMB PRESSURE along the edges of the sacrum, which are the five fused vertebrae that sit just above the coccyx (tailbone). Work on both sides of the sacrum from this side.

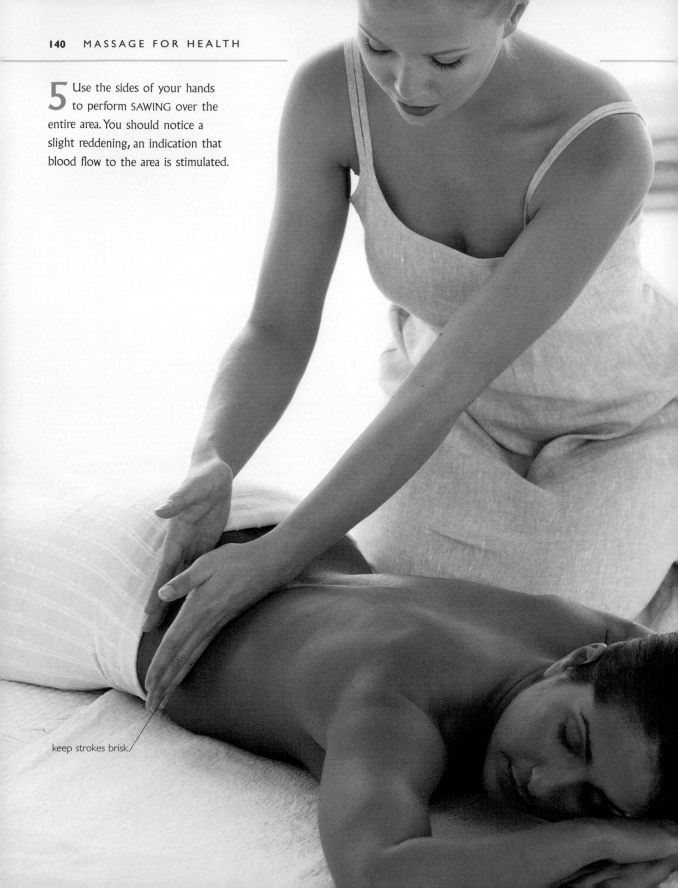

5 Use the sides of your hands to perform SAWING over the entire area. You should notice a slight reddening, an indication that blood flow to the area is stimulated.

keep strokes brisk

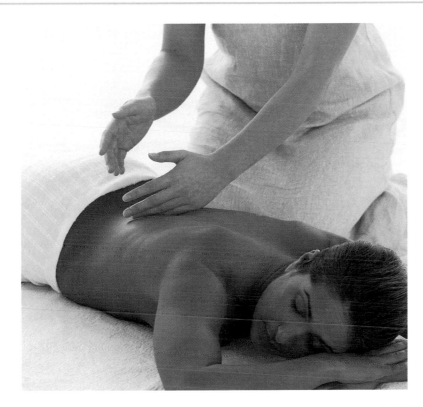

6 Curve your hands slightly, relax your fingers and wrists, and perform HACKING to the lower back and upper part of the buttocks. Maintain a rhythmic pace as you strike the body. This sends vibrations through the area which have a soothing effect.

7 Reach over to work on the opposite side of the back and, keeping your hand flat, perform DEEP LONG STROKING, working from the spine across the muscle fibers. Apply firm pressure, compressing the muscle and "ironing" it out. Then move around and finish the massage by repeating the stroke on the other side of the back.

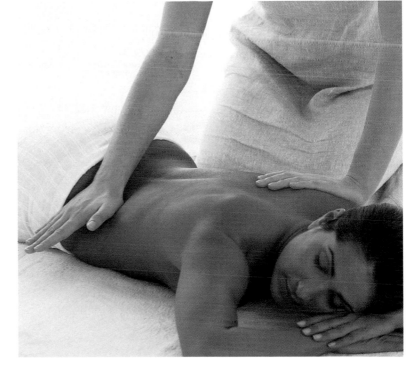

SWEET DREAMS

Slow, rhythmic strokes affect the nervous system, soothing the tension-inducing symptoms of stress by relaxing the muscles and lowering the heart rate. This massage need take no more than 15 minutes and uses no oils or lotions apart from a drop of essential oil behind the ears. I suggest using lavender for its sedative and calming properties. You might also want to make an herb sachet to place under your pillow—the fragrant aromas may help to soothe you to sleep.

TIPS FOR TROUBLED SLEEPERS
If you regularly have trouble sleeping:
• Avoid tea, coffee, or any drink containing caffeine for at least 5 hours before bedtime.
• Take at least 20 minutes of exercise every day.
• Ensure that your bedroom is well-ventilated and not stuffy.
• Don't eat, work, or watch TV in bed.

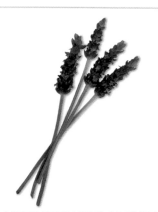

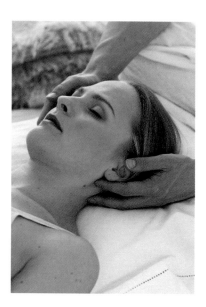

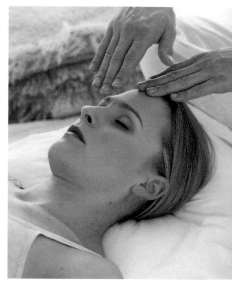

AROMATIC HERB SACHET
◆ I vanilla bean
◆ I sprig fresh or dried lavender
◆ a cotton or linen handkerchief
◆ a length of ribbon or string

Place all of the ingredients in the middle of the handkerchief, and fold to make a sachet. Secure by tying with ribbon or string.

Alternatively, simply put a drop each of vanilla and lavender essential oils on your pillow before you go to bed.

1 Keeping oil away from the eyes, dab one drop of essential oil such as lavender behind each ear. Apply gentle FINGER PRESSURE in small circular movements.

2 Gently stroke the forehead from the eyebrows to the hairline with one hand and then the other in a rhythmic hand-over-hand movement.

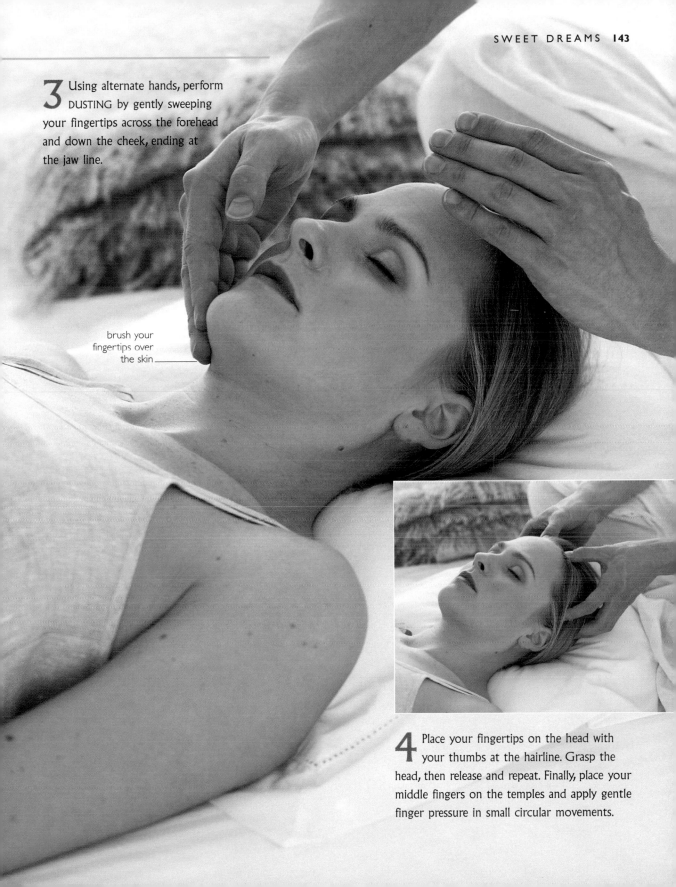

3 Using alternate hands, perform DUSTING by gently sweeping your fingertips across the forehead and down the cheek, ending at the jaw line.

brush your fingertips over the skin

4 Place your fingertips on the head with your thumbs at the hairline. Grasp the head, then release and repeat. Finally, place your middle fingers on the temples and apply gentle finger pressure in small circular movements.

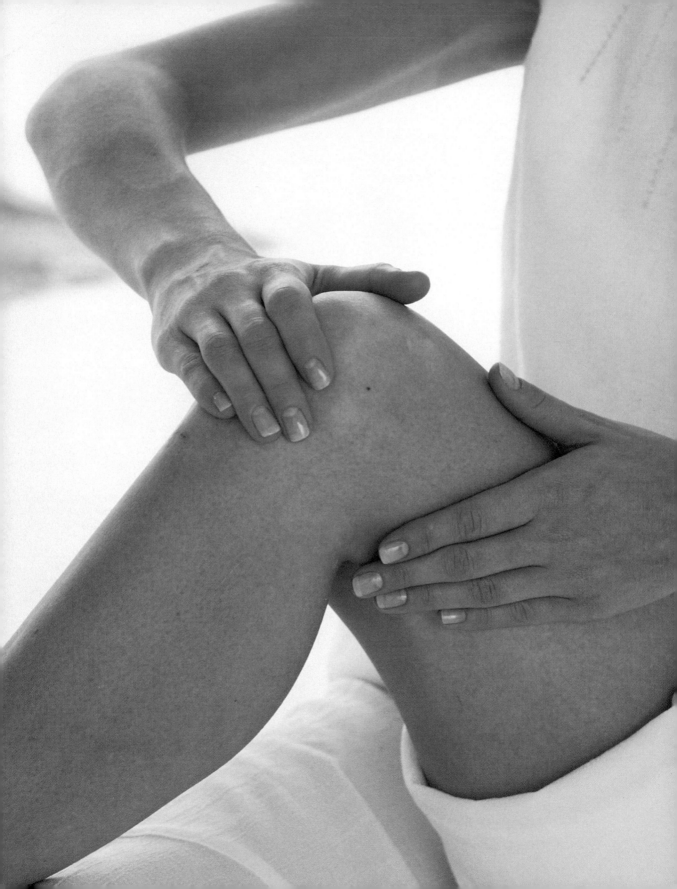

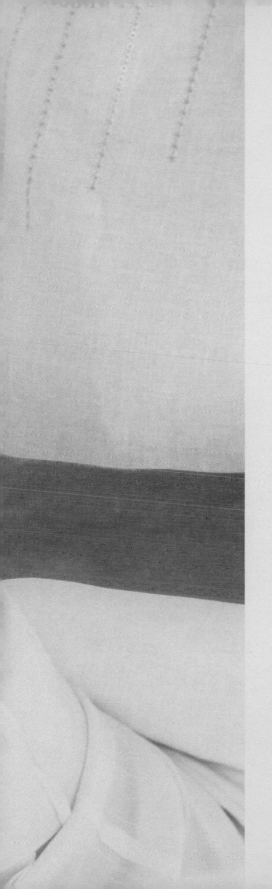

SELF-MASSAGE ROUTINES

I have described how to give an effective and pleasing massage to others, but in the pages that follow you can learn how to soothe and relax your own body by performing simple self-massage. Take the opportunity to experiment with different strokes and to gain an understanding of how your hands feel when massaging other people. The routines that follow will provide relief, but they also give you the excuse to lavish attention on yourself.

SOOTHING TIRED FEET

When you stand or walk, your entire body weight is distributed over a very small surface area—the soles of your feet. Problems with your feet can affect other areas of the body such as the knees and hips. After a long day on your feet, or if you suffer from foot aches or cramps, sit down and take ten minutes to perform this simple routine. It is wonderfully soothing but also restores flexibility, strengthens the muscles in the arch of the foot, and stimulates circulation. Oil or lotion is optional.

MARBLES MASSAGE

Place a handful of marbles together on the floor. Sit in a chair and place one foot on the marbles. Press down gently as you roll your foot over the marbles. This stimulates the reflexology points as well as massaging the many muscles in the sole of the foot.

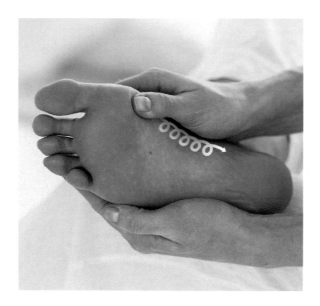

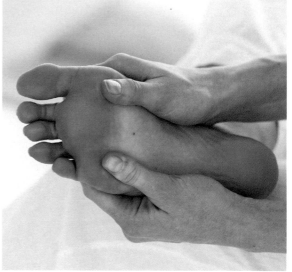

1 Sit down and cross one leg over your knee. Hold your foot in your hand, and with your other hand work around the sole of the foot applying CORKSCREW THUMB PRESSURE in a circular spiralling motion. Work around the foot several times.

2 Cradle your foot in your hands and position your thumbs together just under the toes. Perform THUMB FANNING, gliding your thumbs outward to the edges of the foot and stretching and opening the sole. Repeat, working down the foot.

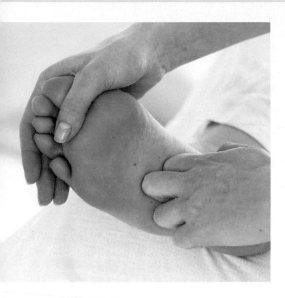

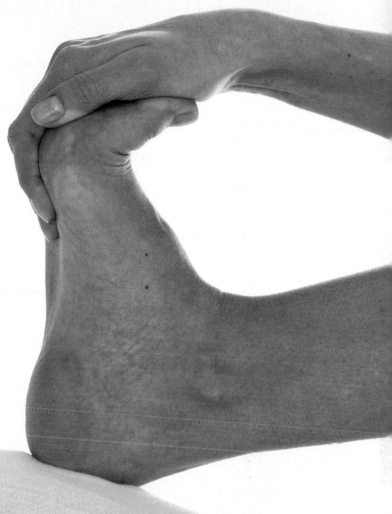

3 Hold the upper part of your foot steady and perform KNUCKLING to the arch. This stretches and strengthens the muscles while also releasing tension.

4 Rest your heel on your knee and take hold of the upper part of your foot. Pull back, bending your toes back and stretching your foot. Release, and repeat several times.

5 Hold your foot with one hand and make a fist with the other. Finish the routine by rapping your knuckles against the sole of your foot. Repeat the entire routine on the other foot.

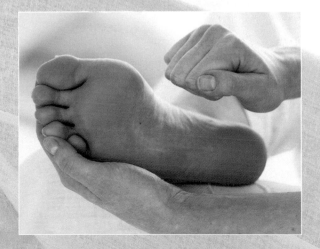

EASING LEG CRAMPS

People who spend a great deal of time on their feet or who wear high heels often complain of leg cramps. This massage can provide immediate relief as it soothes and relaxes the muscles while also boosting circulation. I teach this sequence to clients who frequently travel by plane as maintaining healthy blood circulation in the air can help to prevent deep vein thrombosis. Regular leg massage can also help prevent varicose veins. Perform this massage sitting on the floor or on a chair. Lotion and oil are optional.

PREVENTING LEG CRAMPS
• Take regular exercise, three times a week, to help improve circulation.
• If you have a sedentary job, take regular breaks when you stand up and stretch or go for a short walk.
• If you spend long periods of time on your feet, wear flat shoes that support the arch of the foot.

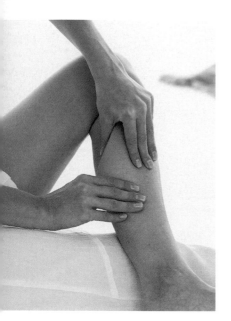

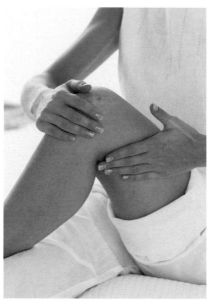

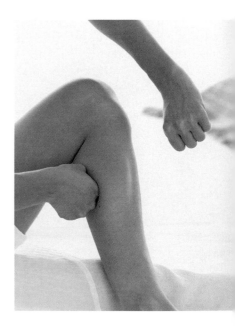

1 Cross one leg over the other. Begin at the top of the calf and use alternate hands to knead down the leg. Grasp and squeeze the muscle with one hand, then release it for the other hand to grasp. Repeat, moving down and up the calf.

2 Place one hand against the front of your knee to keep your leg steady. Starting just above the knee, grasp the flesh between the fingers and thumb of your other hand. Squeeze, then release it and compress it by pressing your hand against your leg. Work up the side of your thigh to the hip.

3 Using alternate hands, perform PUMMELING on one side of your calf and then on the other.

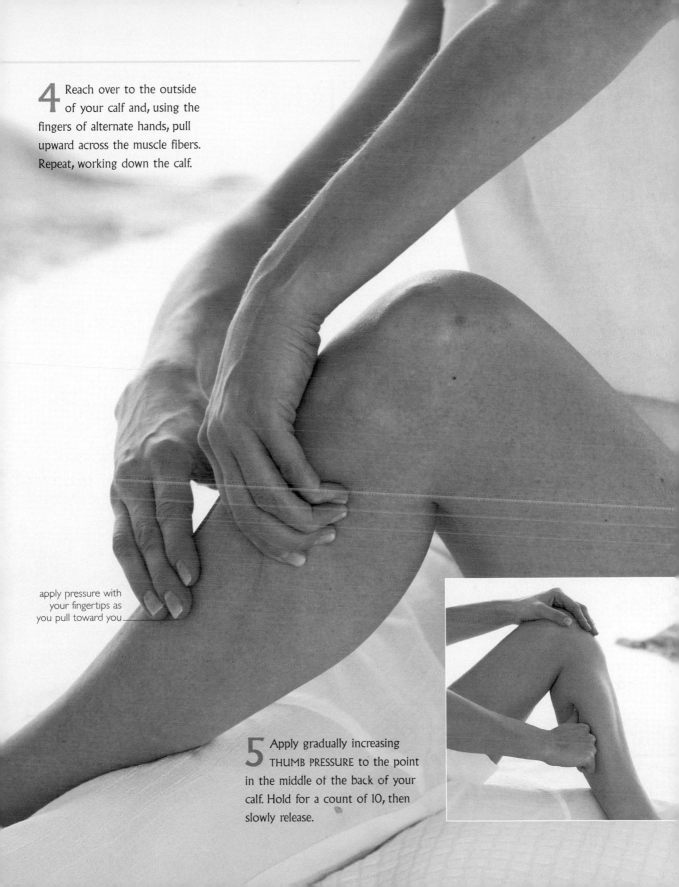

4 Reach over to the outside of your calf and, using the fingers of alternate hands, pull upward across the muscle fibers. Repeat, working down the calf.

apply pressure with
your fingertips as
you pull toward you

5 Apply gradually increasing THUMB PRESSURE to the point in the middle of the back of your calf. Hold for a count of 10, then slowly release.

RELIEF FOR TIRED HANDS

We perform so many actions in everyday life with our hands, it's inevitable that some of the 27 muscles in them will eventually start to feel the strain. If you type regularly or for long periods, it is especially important to stop, give your hands a break, and follow a quick massage routine. If you regularly experience cramps and pains in your hands, you should also regularly practice the pre-massage hand exercises on page 15.

SOOTHING HAND WRAP

In a bowl dissolve ½ a cup of Epsom salts in 3 cups of hot water and add 3 tbsp of witch hazel. Soak a hand towel in the solution, then wring it out and wrap it around your hands. Unwrap after 15 minutes. This boosts circulation and is especially soothing for achy joints.

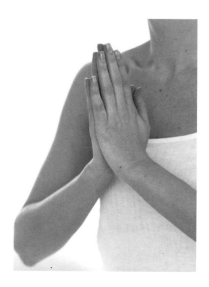

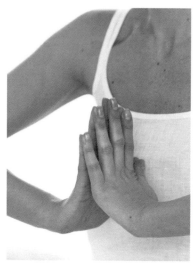

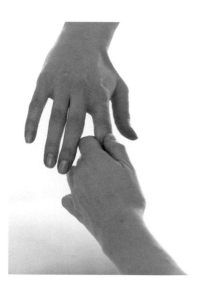

1 Hold your hands at chest height in front of you, with palms pressed together in a praying position. Relax your shoulders.

2 Raise your elbows as you bring your hands down. Feel the stretch in your wrists and in your fingers.

3 Perform TWISTING to each of the sections of your fingers and thumb on one hand and then on the other.

4 Intertwine your fingers with palms facing downward. With your elbows out to your sides, press downward, feeling the stretch in your fingers. Lower your elbows and relax the stretch, then repeat at least 3 times.

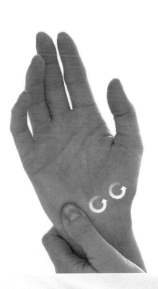

5 Work along the bottom of your palm, applying THUMB PRESSURE in small circular movements. This is a fleshy area so use firm pressure. Repeat on the other hand.

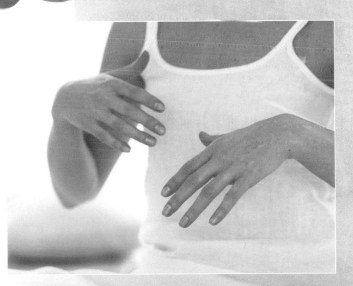

6 Relax your wrists and your fingers, and shake out your hands. Feel your fingers go limp.

BREATHE EASY

If you ever suffer from shortness of breath or a feeling of tightness in the chest as a result of asthma, anxiety, or stress, try this relaxing routine. This massage sequence helps stimulate blood flow to the muscles in the chest, which increases toxin release and enables your ribcage to expand more easily when you breathe. This in turn encourages you to take deeper and more even breaths. The massage can be performed through your clothes or directly on the skin. Oil or lotion is optional.

RELIEVING CONGESTION

Try making this decongestant inhalant at home. The salt makes it portable as it prevents the oils from leaking. Place 2 tsp of salt in a small vial or sealable bag and add one drop each of eucalyptus, peppermint, and rosemary essential oils. Inhale deeply through each nostril to help clear the congestion of a cold or blocked sinuses.

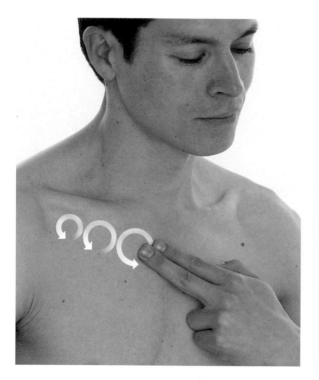

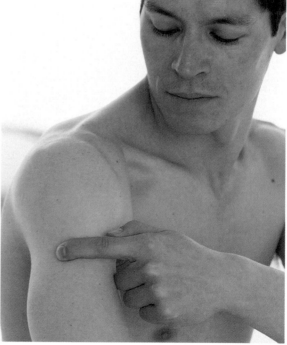

1 Use two fingers to apply FINGER PRESSURE in small circular patterns to the muscles just under your collar bone. Start in the center of your chest and work outward. Repeat, working outward along the collar bone at least 2 more times. Then repeat on the other side.

2 Apply gradually increasing FINGER PRESSURE to the acupressure point on your upper arm (*see above*). Hold for a count of 5, then slowly release. This point stimulates respiratory response. Then repeat at the same point on the other arm.

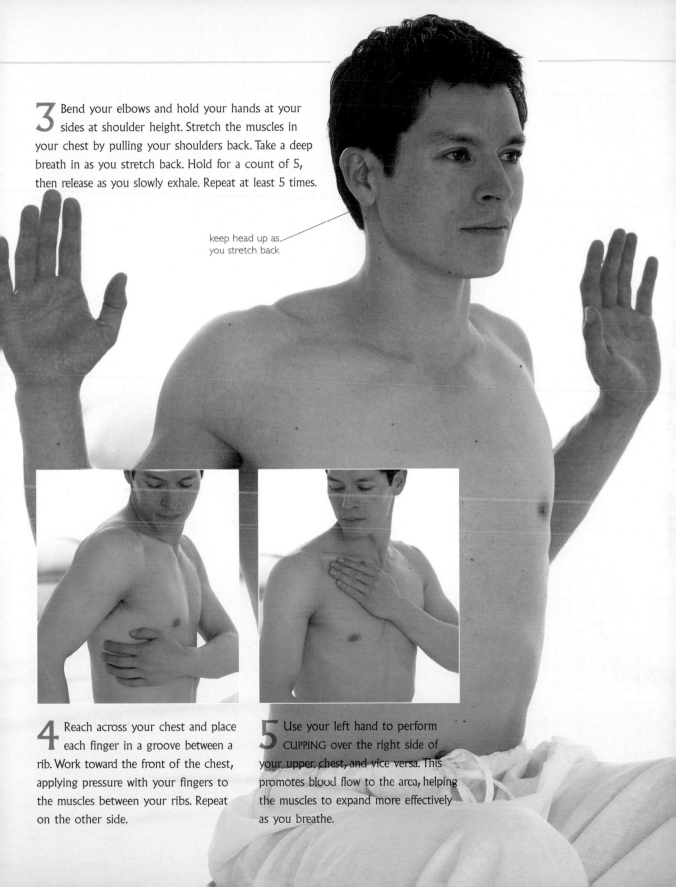

3 Bend your elbows and hold your hands at your sides at shoulder height. Stretch the muscles in your chest by pulling your shoulders back. Take a deep breath in as you stretch back. Hold for a count of 5, then release as you slowly exhale. Repeat at least 5 times.

keep head up as you stretch back

4 Reach across your chest and place each finger in a groove between a rib. Work toward the front of the chest, applying pressure with your fingers to the muscles between your ribs. Repeat on the other side.

5 Use your left hand to perform CUPPING over the right side of your upper chest, and vice versa. This promotes blood flow to the area, helping the muscles to expand more effectively as you breathe.

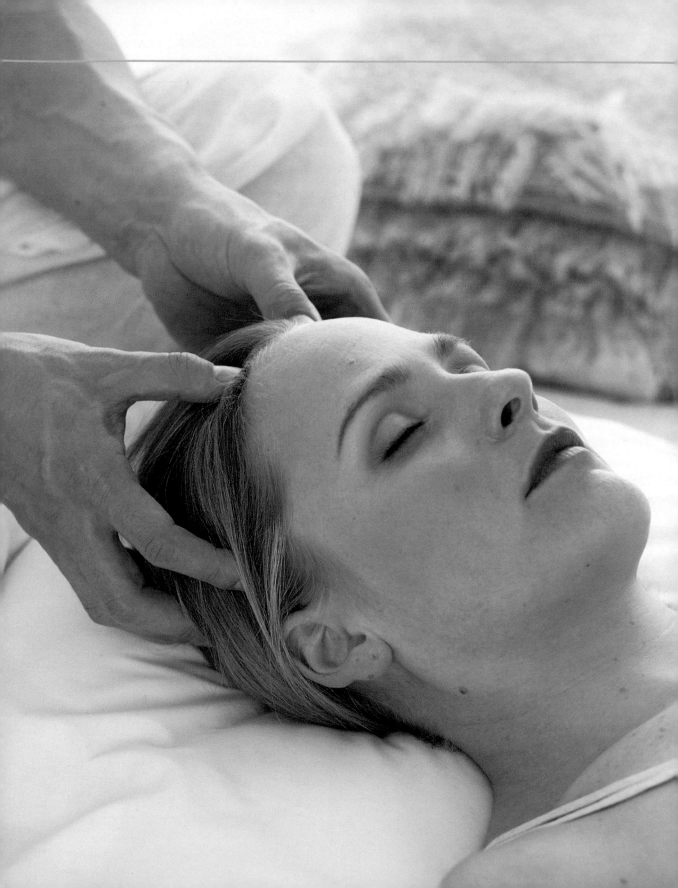

SEEKING EXPERT TREATMENT

Having practiced the strokes and routines in this book, sometimes the best way to improve your technique is to take a few lessons from a professional by simply paying for a session. It's also worth seeking the advice of an experienced professional if you need treatment for a specific muscle complaint or problem. I hope that the information that follows will help you to find a good massage therapist and give you some idea of what to expect during a session.

FINDING A MASSAGE THERAPIST

Personal referrals from friends are the best way to find a massage therapist, but massage schools and associations will also often supply lists of therapists who practice in your area. As massage becomes more widely recognized for its therapeutic benefits, you can expect to find massage therapists working in more varied locations, including: physicians' offices, wellness facilities, chiropractors' offices, rehabilitation clinics, salons, spas, resorts, cruise ships, health clubs, fitness centers, nursing homes, hospitals, the workplace, people's homes, and private practice.

Before embarking on a session, call or ask to meet the therapist first. Ask what types of treatments they offer, and ask them about their training and licensing. It is best to use a massage therapist who has a state, provincial, or national license. Most American states and Canadian provinces now regulate the massage therapy profession by granting licensure to therapists who pass an exam. In the US, licensed therapists abide by the American Massage Therapy Association's code of ethics; in Canada, they are regulated by The Canadian Massage Therapist Alliance.

Even if a therapist is licensed, don't forget to ask for references. Finally, choose a therapist that you like and trust and with whom you feel comfortable. If you don't think you'll feel at ease under his or her hands, it's unlikely you'll relax sufficiently to enjoy— and benefit from—the massage.

DIFFERENT TYPES OF MASSAGE

Remember that there are many different types of massage. The massage that I practice is based on Swedish massage, which uses a combination of stroking, tapping, kneading, and varied pressures to manipulate the muscles. I also incorporate some shiatsu techniques —acupressure massage that follows meridians (pathways) of *chi*, or energy, through the body.

Don't be afraid to ask about what a treatment involves and whether it is suitable for your needs. Remember that each massage therapist will have a different approach to the same treatment, so you may have to try a few therapists before you find one that suits you.

YOUR FIRST MASSAGE

Generally sessions vary in length from 30, 60, 90 to 120 minutes. Sixty minutes is a good length of time for a full body massage; 30 minutes is long enough to address a specific problem.

At the start of the visit, the therapist should ask about your physical fitness. It is your responsibility to provide this information to the best of your knowledge. He or she should also ask what you are hoping to achieve during the treatment. You can request that the therapist concentrate on a particular area, such as the lower back, for the duration of the massage and you can also ask the therapist to avoid any areas that you might not want massaged.

Depending on the therapy, you may have to undress, but you should do what feels comfortable for you. Although most people undress completely for Swedish massage, you can leave your underwear (including your bra) on if you prefer. Some places, like my spa, provide disposable underwear as the oil may mark garments. During the massage, you should be draped at all times, and only the part of the body that is being worked on should be exposed. Some massages, such as shiatsu, office massage, and quick pick-me-up routines, can be performed through clothing.

GETTING THE MOST FROM A SESSION

The most important thing to do is relax. Take deep breaths and entrust yourself to the massage therapist's hands. Look for the following traits in a good masseur:
• a confident touch
• synchronizing breathing with strokes
• ability to feel out sensitive areas
• uses the proper amount of oil
• knowledge of proper draping techniques
• ability to gauge appropriate pressures when performing strokes and movements
• sufficient time spent on each body part.
Let the therapist know if you are unhappy with the music or the temperature in the room, if you want more or less oil, or anything else for that matter. He or she should be happy to oblige.

RIGHT AMOUNT OF PRESSURE

I've been asked before about whether it is acceptable to experience pain during a massage. In fact you have to distinguish between comfortable and uncomfortable pain. When the therapist is working on more sensitive areas, such as knots or lower back pain, he or she should start gently and then gradually begin deeper work. You may experience some discomfort to begin with, but this should diminish after a few minutes as the muscles relax.

This is what I call comfortable pain; you can feel the therapist working with the muscles, not against them. A good therapist should be able to gauge the point at which pain becomes uncomfortable and unpleasant. Pain that causes you to wince, cry out, or tense up is probably not doing you any good. If at any point during the massage, you feel uncomfortable or would prefer lighter or deeper pressure, tell the therapist.

AFTER THE SESSION

When the massage is over, relax for a minute or two and take your time before getting up. You may experience profound relaxation and yet feel strangely invigorated. Some people feel euphoric after a massage. You may feel dizzy or foggy-brained; this occurs as a result of the increased levels of oxygen in your blood from breathing more deeply and from improved circulation. It is also normal to need to urinate after a massage. This is an indication that the process of toxin elimination has been accelerated. Try having a glass of water at the end of the session to help rehydrate you.

In some cases, you may not feel very different until many days after the massage. You may just notice that you feel generally more relaxed and less stressed.

USEFUL RESOURCES

The American Massage Therapy Association
820 Davis Street, Suite 100
Evanston, IL 60201-4444
Tel: (847) 864-0123
Fax: (847) 864-1178
www.amtamassage.org
Represents more than 46,000 massage therapists in 27 countries; works to increase awareness of the benefits of massage; has a nationwide directory of member therapists.

The Touch Research Institute
University of Miami School of Medicine
P.O. Box 016820
Miami Fl 33101
Tel: (305) 243-6781
Fax: (305) 243-6488
Email: tfield@med.miami.edu
www.miami.edu / touch-research
The TRI was the first center in the world devoted solely to the study of touch and its application in science and medicine.

The International Massage Association Group
P.O. Box 421
25 South Fourth Street
Warrenton, VA 20188-0421
Tel: (540) 351-0800
Fax: (540) 351-0816
Email: info@imagroup.com
www.imagroup.com
Provides tools, support, and information for massage and bodywork professionals; works to increase public awareness to the benefits of massage; has a nationwide directory of member therapists.

The Associated Bodywork and Massage Professionals
1271 Sugarbush Drive,
Evergreen, CO 80439-7347
Tel: (800) 458-ABMP (2267)
Fax: (800) 667-8260
Email: expectmore@abmp.com
www.abmp.com
A professional membership association founded in 1987 to provide massage and bodywork practitioners with professional services, information, and public and regulatory advocacy; provides information on the benefits of massage and bodywork. Its current membership is over 38,000.

The Canadian Massage Therapist Alliance
344 Lakeshore Road East
Suite B
Oakville, Ontario L6J 1J6
Canada
Tel: (905) 849-7606
Fax: (905) 849-8606
Email: info@cmta.ca
www.cmta.ca
Fosters and advances the art, science, and philosophy of massage therapy nationwide and represents the different provincial associations; works to increase awareness of the benefits of massage.

INDEX

ACKNOWLEDGMENTS

AUTHOR'S ACKNOWLEDGMENTS

My greatest thanks go to all the people who were involved in putting this book together, especially Nasim Mawji, my editor, Miranda Harvey, who made it look so wonderful, Ruth Jenkinson the photographer, Kerry Lee, her assistant, Stephen McIlmoyle, the make-up artist, Juliet Lee, the stylist, and all of the models. Thanks also to everyone at Dorling Kindersley, particularly Mary-Clare Jerram and also Jenny Lane.

I would also like to thank Mitch Douglas, Sandra Ramani, Dominick Guarnaccia, Paul Selig, the Davidsons, the Semels, and Bobby Driggers.

PUBLISHER'S ACKNOWLEDGMENTS

Dorling Kindersley would like to thank the photographer Ruth Jenkinson and her assistant Kerry Lee, Stephen McIlmoyle, for models' hair and make-up, Juliet Lee for styling, and the models: Abigail Toyne, Belle McLaren, Brigitte Suligoj, Gunilla Johansson, Anton Dean, Ashley Khoo, Sam Whyman, and Rosie Williams. Thanks to Shannon Beatty and Barbara Berger for editorial assistance, and to Sue Bosanko for the index.

Thanks to The White Company (www.whiteco.com, Tel: +44 870 900 9555) for the kind loan of props and models' clothing, and to the Cargo Homeshop (www.cargohomeshop.com, Tel: +44 1844 261 800) for loaning props.

ABOUT THE AUTHOR

Often referred to as "massage therapist to the stars" and once named "best in the city" by American *Vogue,* Larry Costa is one of New York's most sought-after massage therapists. He has acted as consultant on many successful spa projects and owned his own spa, Life is Beautiful, in New York's fashionable SoHo district. Experienced in the fields of chiropractic medical massage and sports massage, Larry spent two years working with the Miami Dolphins' medical team. He has made numerous appearances on US television, including *The Today Show, Live* with Regis and Kathie Lee, and *The View.* Larry has been featured in publications such as *The New York Times, New York* magazine, *Cosmopolitan, Glamour, Allure,* and *Time Out New York.* He lives in New York, where he owns and runs his latest spa venture, The Parlor.